P9-CQN-029

THE

BULLETPROOF DIET

LOSE up to a **POUND** a **DAY,**
RECLAIM Your **ENERGY** and **FOCUS,**
and **UPGRADE** Your **LIFE**

DAVE ASPREY
FOREWORD BY JJ VIRGIN

RODALE.

First published in hardcover by Rodale Inc. in October 2014.

© 2014 by David Asprey

Bulletproof® is a registered trademark of Bulletproof Digital, Inc.

Rodale books may be purchased for business or promotional use or for special sales. For information, e-mail: BookMarketing@gmail.com.

Printed in the United States of America

Rodale Inc. makes every effort to use acid-free ♾, recycled paper ♻.

Book design by Joanna Williams

Library of Congress Cataloging-in-Publication Data is on file with the publisher.

ISBN 978–1–62336–518–9   hardcover
ISBN 978–1–62336–838–8   paperback

Distributed to the trade by Macmillan

10   9   hardcover
8   10   9   7   paperback

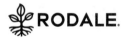

We inspire and enable people to improve their lives and the world around them.
rodalebooks.com

To my kids, Anna and Alan.

May you grow up in a world full of happy people who eat real food that makes them thrive. Then hack it even more.

CONTENTS

FOREWORD

Dave Asprey might be the most inspirational biohacker I know. He hacked his own body to achieve a new kind of physical and mental clarity, and his story empowers others to take control over their health. He did this through herculean trial-and-error to develop a system that helped him lose over 100 pounds. Today he's got not only a six-pack, but also amazing mental acuity and physical vigor.

Using your body as a chemistry lab to connect what you're eating and how you feel—in other words, becoming a biohacker—might be the most powerful thing you can do for fat loss and optimal health. I've long argued your body is a chemistry lab, not a bank account. The calories-in-calories-out weight loss model has devolved into a nutrition dinosaur because while calories matter, hormones count more. Food is information, not a math equation.

Take gluten. You've probably read about its potential problems and how a well-designed gluten-free diet can become beneficial. Yet a complete incentive to change can only occur when you directly connect those effects with how they adversely impact your life. Rather than scold yourself for eating something bad, feeling your fingers swell and seeing your skin break out provide an entirely new understanding about how gluten impacts your body. Dave's goal was to figure out how and why these things were happening to him, and to fix them for good.

My gateway to Dave's world, probably like yours, involved a special kind of toxin-free upgraded coffee. Coffee gets me excited. I've long considered it a health food, and if I could classify it as a food group it would quickly become my favorite. Yet something about conventional coffee always left me feeling jittery. I would become buzzed out and then crash hard.

Then I heard Dave talk about how mycotoxins, or mold toxins, became the Kryptonite that created this crash. Also a stalwart coffee lover, Dave created a special blend of beans that eliminated those nasty contaminants. All that sounded well and good, but I became especially intrigued when I heard he added grass-fed butter to his coffee. Surely I'm not the only one who initially remarked, "Butter in coffee: *Really*?"

From my understanding, Dave got this idea from a Himalayan hike, where he enjoyed tea blended and yak butter. He played around with a coffee variation until he created what we now call Bulletproof Coffee, which gives you this beloved beverage's boost without a subsequent crash.

Dave actually made me my first cup. The hot, creamy, decadent drink tasted fabulous and curbed my hunger for hours. You mean I could drink this stuff every morning and *burn* fat? Plus, these seemingly magical beans gave me improved mental clarity and a newfound energy with none of conventional coffee's adverse effects.

Today I serve Bulletproof Coffee at all my events, and make sure I have enough during conferences and anywhere I need to be alert and focused for hours. I've even had colleagues remark, "How did we function before Bulletproof Coffee?"

Bulletproof Coffee is amazing, but Dave has even more biohacks up his sleeve. Dave also designed an intelligent, cutting-edge plan based on his own transformation that optimizes hormones, improves mental clarity, and makes you an all-day fat burner. For busy professionals, this plan became a no-brainer: Simply enjoy satiating Bulletproof Coffee for breakfast and then two satisfying, nutrient-dense meals. Couldn't be easier.

With *The Bulletproof Diet*, you too can utilize that peak-performance plan to become lean, healthy, and mentally focused. This groundbreaking book provides a simple-to-follow roadmap that addresses food intolerances and other potential difficulties, creates hormonal balance, and leaves you performing like a rock star.

Food forms the forefront of the Bulletproof plan. The Bulletproof Roadmap, as Dave calls it, provides a dietary guide that tastes good, edges out the bad stuff, destroys cravings, and helps you feel better so you kick more ass. That Roadmap removes any guesswork out of what foods to enjoy, limit, and eliminate. Many might surprise you, especially if you thought fruit was healthy or particular oils can become artery clogging.

Speaking of misconceptions, *The Bulletproof Diet* dispels plenty of conventional, outdated, or just downright incorrect nutrition myths that hold your health hostage. In Dave's book you'll learn how dietary fat can help you become lean, that you don't need to count calories to burn fat, how fruit can stall fat loss, and why you shouldn't graze throughout the day.

Totally contrary to what you've long heard, right? Some of Dave's advice might even initially seem a little crazy. Dave also makes a pretty bold claim you'll benefit from right away on the plan: "Lose a Pound a Day Without Being Hungry" during your first two weeks. Who doesn't want that?

To get those results, you needn't starve yourself or spend hours in the gym. (You'll actually learn in this book why those things could work against you.) Instead, you'll lower inflammation, boost your sex drive, turn back the clock, and ditch that stubborn weight with the power of your fork and the right coffee.

Altogether, *The Bulletproof Diet* weaves together a battle-tested plan that gets results, even if (*especially* if) past eating plans failed you. *The Bulletproof Diet* provides a solid, well-designed, easy-to-follow plan to efficiently, effortlessly burn fat, perform like a rock star, and reach a new level of amazing. Who knew a simple cup of coffee could become the foundation for all that?

—JJ Virgin, *New York Times* bestselling author of *The Virgin Diet*, *The Virgin Diet Cookbook*, and *The Sugar Impact Diet*

⬤ INTRODUCTION

THE BULLETPROOF EXECUTIVE

Nearly 2 decades ago, I was a young, brand-new multimillionaire entre-preneur in Silicon Valley. Life should have been awesome, but there was one problem—I was obese, weighing in at almost 300 pounds. For 18 months straight, I had tried restricting my eating to 1,500 to 1,800 calories a day and working out for 90 minutes, six times a week. I poured my initiative and willpower into losing weight, and while I did get stronger, the extra fat wouldn't go away. By the time I was 30, I was diag-nosed with the rapid onset of second-phase thrombin-induced platelet aggregation. Basically, my blood was thick, like sludge, and my physician was concerned that I would die of a stroke or heart attack—not at some indeterminate time in the future, but soon.

Despite my career success, most of the time I felt too awful to appreci-ate it. I was always tired and consumed by stress, and I was sick all of the time with chronic sinus infections and strep throat. My brain felt foggy, and I had trouble focusing. When I was getting my MBA at the Wharton School of the University of Pennsylvania while also working at a startup, my performance on exams was horrible. I'd get a couple questions right, and then despite my best efforts, I'd make unconscious mistakes on the rest. It felt like something in my brain was betraying me. I knew how to do the work, but when I really tried to concentrate I just couldn't "bring it."

This was frightening. Being fat was bad enough, but if I was going to be fat and also be stupid, there was no way I could make a living doing the work I love. This motivated me to research the latest brain imaging techniques, and I finally decided to undergo a then-controversial technique called a single-photon emission computed tomography (SPECT) scan so I could finally learn why my brain was betraying me. On the appointed day at Silicon Valley Brain Imaging, a technician injected radioactive sugar into my arm. My brain then used the sugar, and a radioactive tracer revealed that in my prefrontal cortex—the most advanced, recently evolved part of the brain—there was essentially no activity when I tried to concentrate. I was losing not only my health in what should have been the prime of my life, but also experiencing failure of my brain's basic "hardware." The worst part was that I didn't understand why this was happening. After all, I was doing everything that my doctors and all mainstream medical professionals were telling me to do.

I grew up in the world of hard science, and this has informed the way I look at problem solving. My grandparents met on the Manhattan Project and my grandmother won a prestigious lifetime achievement award for her work in nuclear science. Since I got my own computer at age 8, I'm also one of the few 40-somethings who's been working with computers for more than 30 years. My undergraduate concentration was in decision support systems, a specialty within the field of artificial intelligence. The power of science and technology has been a part of my life for as long as I can remember, and when faced with a health and career crisis, I turned to this power to try and find some answers.

I was an early innovator in the Internet (i.e., a hacker), and before attending Wharton I ran an instructional program at the University of California extension offices in Silicon Valley. From 1997 to 2002 I taught engineers there how to manage the Internet. This was notoriously hard to do back then because engineers (like medical specialists) like to know every bit of data about the system they're working with, and it just wasn't available then. With the Internet, you often have to "make it go" even when you don't have the luxury of seeing what all of the pieces involved are doing. In this way, our bodies and the Internet are not all that different. They are both complex systems with big pieces of data that are missing, misunderstood, or hidden. When I looked at my body that way, I realized that I could learn to hack my biology using the same techniques I used to hack computer systems and the Internet.

This was a major turning point and the beginning of my journey into biohacking—the art of using technology to change the environment both inside and outside of your body to take control and make it do what you want. I was excited by the idea of monitoring my own health to uncover the hidden variables that were affecting how I felt, how I looked, how I performed, and even my relationships and overall happiness. Computer hackers map out a computer system and then attempt to find one little hole they can exploit in order to take over, often by trying each potential flaw until finding the one that lets them in. This is the same process that makes biohacking work. I started to measure my physical output and experiment with my body to troubleshoot the world around me and see what was influencing my performance. Nothing was too "out there" or too small. I got my blood chemistry done and measured my stress levels through adrenal hormone testing. After compiling the results, I started using "smart drugs" to turn my brain back on, adding supplements, and experimenting with countless diets to see what worked, what didn't, and why.

Since then, I've explored private brain-hacking facilities hidden in the Canadian forest, spiritual practices in the Andes, and remote monasteries in Tibet. I installed an electroencephalogram (EEG) brain-wave monitoring machine in my home office and became certified in using a biofeedback technique called heart rate variability to learn how to control my nervous system's stress response. As I used these techniques to master my brain, it became clear that what I ate had a direct impact on my biology and my thinking. When my biology changed, my mental and physical performance did, too. Using these devices to monitor my brain allowed me to see which foods improved my mental performance and which ones destroyed it.

This was the genesis of the Bulletproof Diet. By experimenting with so many different variables, correlating the feedback, and peeling back layer after layer of the available research, I learned about the complex roles that inflammation, toxins, hormones, neurotransmitters, gut bacteria, and many other factors play when it comes to weight loss, hunger, and energy levels. Lots of these discoveries are in obscure research journals and haven't been widely used, and others are the result of my own careful observations, and observations shared by other biohackers. These findings were surprising, but they allowed me to lose weight at the rate of up to a pound a day and look better than ever while gaining amazing levels of performance, resilience, and focus. I learned how to fuel my body and my brain properly and, just as important, to rid my life of the things that were secretly holding me back.

My results were so counterintuitive that at first I thought it was just me. Perhaps there was something odd about the way my personal biochemistry responded to food. But as I shared my discoveries with friends and family members and saw them rapidly losing weight, too, while also increasing their mental focus and gaining willpower, I knew I was onto something. Now it's your turn to benefit from my years of research and experimentation. By following the Bulletproof Diet, you'll be able to lose weight, improve your overall performance, and gain an edge on life through increased energy and resilience. For more than a decade now, I have maintained a 100-pound weight loss and even grown a six-pack while lowering my biological age and turbocharging my immune system. My 40s are truly better than my 20s, and yours can be, too.

The truth is that although I say I've lost 100 pounds, I've actually lost far more than that, because every time I tried a new diet I lost a bunch of weight and then ended up gaining it back and then some. Then I'd move on to the next diet, lose weight, and gain it back again. Low-calorie diets, high-protein diets, low-fat diets, liquid diets, Zone, Atkins—I tried them all, even spending almost a year on a raw vegan diet. This cycle continued for years, as I gained and lost the same weight over and over again, all the while monitoring how each diet influenced my energy, mood, and cravings.

If you're overweight, does this sound familiar? Do you have a pair of "fat jeans" hiding in your closet because deep down you know that no matter how many diets you try, you'll always need them again once you run out of willpower, "fall off the wagon," and then feel guilty for eating the pizza you told yourself you weren't going to eat? For years my fat jeans sat in my closet just waiting for me to fail again. They had a 46-inch waist.

It wasn't until I hacked the Bulletproof Diet that I was able to finally throw those jeans out for good and stop wasting my willpower on food. And now you'll be able to get rid of your fat jeans, too, as you start kicking ass, losing weight, and living up to your full potential.

Chances are that if you picked up this book, you're not just looking to lose a few pounds. Your life is stressful, and you also want to improve your performance while experiencing easy and sustained weight loss that feels great and tastes even better. Imagine trying to negotiate a business agreement, staying up all night with a sick kid, and then focusing at work the next day, or attempting to think of a new solution to a complex problem when you're fighting food cravings and your body feels like it's been inside a cement mixer for a few days. If you're like me, your life is a tour de force, or maybe you just want it to be. Looking and *feeling* sick, tired, fat, or weak is not an option, and you were not meant to be that way.

We live in a fast-paced world where so many people waste time feeling sluggish and confused, wanting to look, feel, and perform better but not knowing how or understanding why it's not happening for them. They imagine it's because they simply lack the willpower or don't try hard enough. The Bulletproof Diet is the antidote to all of this. It's not just about losing weight fast and feeling fantastic; it's a roadmap to upgrading your body and your mind from the inside out, simultaneously suppressing the inflammation and guilt that often come with high stress, high expectations, and high performance. On the Bulletproof Diet, guilt is a thing of the past. Most people feel guilty when they have a food craving, but biohackers look

The Bulletproof Diet isn't just about losing weight fast and feeling fantastic; it's a roadmap to upgrading your body and your mind from the inside out, simultaneously suppressing the inflammation and guilt that often come with high stress, high expectations, and high performance.

for the environmental trigger that might have been the cause. The Bulletproof Diet works to remove these potential triggers so you'll never have to waste time feeling guilty about food again.

My personal experience has been reinforced by a decade of leadership in the antiaging field as president, chairman, or a board member of the Silicon Valley Health Institute. There, I've had the opportunity to host conversations with more than 100 top medical professionals and researchers, and I've learned from more than 100 other top experts in human performance on my number one–ranked health podcast and nationally syndicated radio show, *Bulletproof Radio*. The information in this book is based on the distilled knowledge of those experts and the results of the more than $300,000 I spent biohacking myself with self-experiments.

For you, becoming Bulletproof might mean having more energy on less sleep, losing weight with minimal exercise, or simply feeling like the lights in your brain have turned on for the first time and you finally have the power to be your most awesome, powerful self. What will you be capable of when you're no longer distracted by hunger, energy crashes, or food cravings? Whether you're a superstar, an entrepreneur, or a busy mom or dad who needs to do more in less time, this is your chance to find out. Throughout the book I've included personal stories and anecdotes that illustrate how the Bulletproof Diet has worked for me, but you can ignore those entirely as you learn to customize it so that *you* operate at your optimal level. Remember, you're the one who matters, and what works for one person—including me—may not be the precise formula for you, but the core principles are the same!

I'm not the only one to have benefited from the Bulletproof Diet. In my thriving consulting practice, I use the information in this book to help celebrities, athletes, entrepreneurs, CEOs, professional poker players, and hedge fund managers perform at the very top of their fields, where a tiny boost in performance can make the difference between winning and losing. Elite athletes, fitness models, Hollywood celebrities, and Billboard artists have also turned to the Bulletproof Diet to achieve ultimate focus and energy along with camera-ready looks. Online, more than 50,000 people are using the Bulletproof Diet principles to realize the same life-changing weight loss and performance enhancement that my consulting clients and I have, and the results they've shared are spectacular—amazing energy levels and improved brain power along with weight loss, often at a rate of 1 pound per day for sustained periods of time.

You may be surprised to realize that your diet has so much to do with your mental and physical performance, and at first I was, too. The truth is that there are many elements of your environment that affect your performance, but there is no more powerful variable than your diet when you're trying to control your body to get the outcome you desire. Even exercise pales in comparison. This may seem like hyperbole, but your diet is the foundation behind not only your weight, but also your IQ, stress levels, risk of disease, physical performance, aging, and even willpower. You *are* what you eat. What would it feel like to improve in all of these areas simply by making better choices about what you put on your plate? When you begin following the Bulletproof Diet, you'll know the answer within only 2 weeks while losing up to a pound a day and never feeling deprived or hungry. Are you ready to become Bulletproof and start living in a constant state of high performance? Let's get started!

CHAPTER

1

BIOHACK YOUR DIET TO LOSE WEIGHT AND UPGRADE YOUR LIFE

B ack when I was fat, I'd wake up with my hands noticeably weaker on some days than others. Looking in the mirror, I would see puffiness around my face and jawline. I had multiple chins, and, most embarrassingly, I had grown a nice set of man boobs that could go up or down nearly a cup size from one day to the next. Sure, these are all symptoms of being overweight, but I didn't understand why they were so much worse on some days than on others. Within a few days I'd lose or gain a few pounds and even notice a huge difference in the size of the spare tire around my waist.

The very act of noticing these things motivated me to find out what factors in my environment might be causing them. A nagging voice in my head asked, "If something is making your hands weak, what else is it doing?" I started researching possible causes and found that my weak

1

hands, spare tire, double chin, puffy skin, and even my man boobs weren't made of fat—they were signs of inflammation. (Granted, there was plenty of fat hiding underneath the inflammation!) As an antiaging biohacker, I knew that inflammation is a major cause of aging, but I hadn't realized that nearly everything else happening to my biology was related to inflammation, too.

For years, if I took a short walk, I'd often end up with blisters on my feet. The walk to the school where I was getting my MBA was only a quarter of a mile, but on some days I'd show up to class limping with fresh blisters. My research told me that blisters were a sign of chronic inflammation and that brain fog—grasping for words and slow recall—can be a symptom of brain inflammation. It seemed that I had found the missing link between my physical and mental performance that had eluded me for years. When I finally hacked inflammation, I was able to trek across the Himalayas in Nepal and Tibet without blisters for the first time in my life, and my brain worked better, too.

Inflammation is the body's natural response to a pathogen, toxin, stress, or trauma. When something stresses the body, it responds by swelling up in an effort to heal itself. Inflammation is necessary for proper tissue repair. You get healthy inflammation after you lift weights and your body works to repair the stressed muscle or when you cut yourself and increased blood flow ferries in white blood cells to heal the injury. This is called acute inflammation, and if you've ever had an injury or surgery, you've seen firsthand how the body can swell during times of physical stress. It's when inflammation becomes chronic (lasting for months or years) that it causes serious problems. Imagine if you had knee surgery or a root canal and the swelling and puffiness never calmed down. You don't look or feel good when you're carrying around excess inflammation, and doing so is actually quite dangerous.

Research has shown time and again that high levels of inflammation are at the center of many diseases. Together, cardiovascular diseases, various cancers, and diabetes account for almost 70 percent of all deaths in the United States, and the common link between all of these diseases is inflammation[1,2] Inflammation is also linked to many autoimmune diseases and some mental health issues.[3] It's an insidious condition, because, like me, you likely don't feel the extent of it, and it saps your focus because your brain is exquisitely sensitive to inflammation anywhere in the body. Unchecked inflammation takes away your mental edge long before it causes you to feel physical pain or discomfort. That's right: Treat your brain fog or constant bloat now because they can be warning signs of more serious problems down the line.

I realized that inflammation was limiting my physical performance and to some extent my mental performance, too. But what was causing all this inflammation? I began studying causes of inflammation and found a huge body of research on the abundant antinutrients in most standard diets that can cause chronic inflammation. They do this by irritating the gut, which triggers the immune system, or otherwise damaging the body's repair and detoxification systems. The body responds as if it's been injured and becomes inflamed in an effort to heal. Then it gets even worse—your irritated intestinal lining allows undigested food particles and bacteria to enter your bloodstream and trigger a wider inflammatory response as your body attacks these foreign particles. When these antinutrients continually damage your gut, which unfortunately happens to most people on Western diets that include large amounts of inflammation-causing processed foods, your body is forced to constantly mount a response against a perceived enemy. It does this by releasing a stream of small inflammatory proteins called cytokines into your bloodstream, which eventually enter your brain. An inflamed brain is an unhappy, low-performance brain that will make you act like a jerk even when you don't want to.

Antinutrients play a much bigger role in how you feel every day than you might imagine. They can be a source of severe food cravings that distract you from whatever you're trying to accomplish, or they can rob you of nutrients and interfere with your hormone function, wearing down different systems in your body and causing slow performance declines over time. Depending on the severity of antinutrient exposure and your genetics, your body may mount an autoimmune reaction. This causes even more damage as your immune system attacks important body systems.[4]

The trick is to reduce your body's immune response by eating fewer foods with antinutrients and avoiding entirely the foods that trigger your immune system. Most people are aware of toxins, one form of antinutrients that may be added to food, such as preservatives, pesticides, or colorings, but few understand that those toxins can cause food cravings and diminish mental performance. Even fewer people are aware of naturally occurring antinutrients that are hidden sources of Kryptonite in your daily life. These toxins form in plants and plant products as they are growing or in storage, and their main function is to keep animals, bugs, and fungi from eating the plants so the plants can reproduce. That's right—plants did not evolve for us to eat them; they evolved complex defense systems to *keep* us from eating them!

By avoiding these nutritional landmines, your body and mind will be able to function at their best so you can feel what it's like to be in the Bulletproof state of high performance. Don't get me wrong; humans have survived for generations eating foods that are high in antinutrients. But the goal of the Bulletproof Diet is the opposite of surviving—it is thriving.

The main categories of naturally occurring antinutrients are lectins, phytates, oxalates, and mold toxins (mycotoxins).

LECTINS

A lectin is a type of protein that permanently attaches itself to the sugars that line your cells, disrupting small-intestine metabolism and damaging gut villi (fingerlike projections on the small intestine's lining that absorb nutrients) or even your joints. There are thousands of types of lectins, and they are part of most life-forms. Not all of them are toxic or cause intestinal damage. The lectins we're talking about are specific compounds made by plants that bind to joints, irritate the gut, lead to bacterial overgrowth, and contribute to leptin (with a *p*!) resistance, a condition that causes the brain of an overweight person not to receive the signal that the stomach is full.[5] A few of these antinutrients are found in lots of plant and animal foods, but certain plants such as beans, nuts, and grains contain dramatically higher levels than others. The more of those lectins you consume, the more you risk damaging your body, and there is no benefit to choosing high-lectin foods.

Certain people are more sensitive to specific types of lectins than others. If you eat something that contains the type of lectins you're sensitive to (or a lot of lectins that you're somewhat less sensitive to), the result is inflammation that you may experience as brain fog, sore joints, bad skin, or even migraines. For example, the type of lectins found in the nightshade family of plants, which includes tomatoes, eggplants, peppers, and potatoes, is one that many people are sensitive to. It is a common autoimmune trigger that has been linked to a significant percentage of rheumatoid arthritis cases and is a trigger for skin problems.

Luckily, *most* lectins are destroyed by heat and can be reduced or eliminated by using certain cooking methods. But there are some foods, including the nightshade family of vegetables, whose lectins are not destroyed by heat. The Bulletproof Diet helps you steer clear of the problems caused by lectins by having you eat fewer of the high-lectin foods. Once you're in maintenance mode, you can test yourself to see how you feel with or without specific high-lectin foods in your diet. The goal is to personalize your diet to provide the most flexibility and the most energy and focus.

PHYTATES

Phytates are another plant defense system evolved to prevent animals and insects from eating them. They function by binding to dietary minerals that animals need to be healthy, particularly iron, zinc, magnesium, and calcium. This slows or prevents the minerals' absorption[6] so you get little nutrition from the food. Whole grains, nuts, and seeds are the major sources of these antinutrients. Phytates are actually antioxidants, molecules that prevent other molecules from becoming oxidized or damaged. Consuming antioxidants is normally a good thing, but some antioxidants, like phytates, have both negative and positive effects. Your body can handle a certain amount of phytates, and eliminating them from your diet completely wouldn't be possible, but it's a good idea to minimize the main sources so your minerals will be absorbed.

Cooking certain foods that are high in phytates and then draining the water or soaking them in something acidic like lemon or vinegar minimizes phytates, but many of the grains and seeds that contain phytates are irritating to the gut even when cooked. Certain animals like cows and sheep have special bacteria in their guts to help them break down phytates. Humans, pigs, and chickens don't have this bacteria. This is one reason it's best to avoid most direct sources of phytates and eat more grass-fed cows and sheep, allowing them to filter out the phytates for you. This way you get the benefits of foods that contain phytates without the toxins.

OXALATES

Oxalic acid (oxalates) is another antinutrient that forms in plants to protect them from predation by animals, insects, and fungi. They're found in raw cruciferous vegetables such as kale, chard, and spinach, as well as buckwheat, black pepper, parsley, poppy seeds, rhubarb, amaranth, beets, chocolate, most nuts, most berries, and beans.

When oxalates bind to calcium in your blood, tiny, sharp oxalic acid crystals form and can be deposited anywhere in the body and cause muscle pain. When this happens in the kidneys, it is one cause of kidney stones. It sounds hard to believe, but oxalates also cause painful sex in some women when oxalic acid crystals form in the labia. Before my wife, Lana, went Bulletproof, she suffered greatly from this oxalic acid–related condition, called vulvodynia, the cause of which is considered a mystery by Western medicine, with theorized links to yeast problems, antibiotic use, and emotional issues. For sensitive people, consuming even a small amount of oxalates can cause burning in the mouth, eyes, ears, and throat. Larger doses can lead to muscle weakness, abdominal pain, nausea, vomiting, and diarrhea, especially in people with a high body burden of oxalates. In my time as a raw vegan eating tons of raw kale, broccoli, and chard, I experienced oxalate-related weakness that was hard to explain until I understood this.

As with phytates, soaking in acid or cooking *and draining away the cooking water* minimizes oxalates, so I don't recommend eating raw kale, spinach, or chard in salads or even smoothies. It's also important to choose your nuts and chocolate carefully, and I'll guide you through this in great detail later in the book. Quality matters more than you'd think!

MOLD TOXINS

The final major class of antinutrients in your diet is mold toxins (mycotoxins). Most people are exposed to chronic low doses of mold toxins in every single meal, but they are invisible and particularly hard to identify. The more mold toxins you eat, the more damage they do over time. I probably never would have recognized this if it weren't for my familiarity with toxic mold.

Both as a kid and later as an adult, I unknowingly lived in several moldy houses. Because of the repeated exposures, my immune system is more sensitive than the average person's to mold in my environment or in my food. On a business trip to the United Kingdom, I once went down into the Tube and noticed the dank air. By the time I reached the end of the passenger tunnel and got on the train, I started to feel like I was hungover and even had some visual hallucinations. That's how sensitive I am to mold. Right after that experience, I had profound cravings for sugar and fat, and it took almost a full day before it felt like my brain had turned back on. My meetings later that day in Cambridge didn't go so well, but my extreme reaction to mold has been a blessing in disguise. It has enabled me to help clients identify why they have seemingly inexplicable declines in mental and physical performance and led me to learn more about the biochemistry of mold exposure both in sensitive people like me (about 28 percent of the population), and in the rest of us. If you're not feeling amazing, there is always a reason!

I've known for a long time that being in a moldy environment was awful for cognitive performance, but it was coffee that first turned me on to mold toxins in food. Coffee has been a great passion of mine since I first discovered that it improved my grades in college. While studying computer science, I was forced to sign up for an 8:00 a.m. calculus class. Being the opposite of a morning person, I ventured into the world of triple espresso shots before class and earned the only A I ever got in 2 years of studying calculus. I was hooked, and I soon launched my first entrepre-neurial venture, which was inadvertently the first example of e-commerce

I used to drink corporate coffee every day and would notice a dip in energy 3 to 4 hours after drinking just one cup of black iced coffee. Since switching to Bulletproof Coffee with butter and MCT oil, my days are full of energy—and I'm pretty sure I cured a mild case of adrenal fatigue. Incredible! —**Colin** in history. It was fueled by coffee, just as all good entrepreneurial ventures seem to be these days. I created and sold a T-shirt over the Internet (before we had Web browsers even!) that said "Caffeine: My drug of choice," along with a picture of the caffeine molecule. Twenty years later, you can still buy knockoffs of that design online.

Imagine my dismay a few years later when I began to notice that coffee wasn't serving me. I'd drink it, get a boost, and then start to feel fatigued and cranky, like I needed more coffee. I was constantly upping my dose, which sometimes led to headaches. Wanting to rid myself of these symptoms, I gave up the black brew for 5 long, dark years. One day, coffee's siren call was strong enough to compel me to have "just one cup," and I felt amazing. No crash. No jitters. No headache. Just pure focus, the way I remembered. I was elated that coffee appeared to no longer be a problem for me.

What happened the next day is a part of the reason this book exists. I had another cup of coffee, and this time I felt anxious and weak, and later my joints hurt—totally not Bulletproof. But this time the biohacker in me realized that the key variable wasn't me; it was the coffee! I dug into the biochemistry of coffee and the agricultural and economic research to discover that all coffee is not the same, and that coffee often carries naturally occurring mold toxins. It turned out that my reaction to certain coffees had nothing to do with the coffee; it was a reaction to the *mold* on the coffee.

When exposed to even low levels of mold toxins, many people lose their edge. At higher levels, mold toxins cause serious damage, such as cardiomyopathy, cancer, hypertension, kidney disease, and even brain damage. Coffee can taste bitter (like it needs sugar) when it's roasted wrong, or when the coffee plant experiences unhealthy stressors, including pathogenic fungi.

The amount of mold on coffee beans can even vary from batch to batch, especially for large coffee producers. Mold toxins are present in a significant amount of coffee. One study testing green coffee beans grown in Brazil showed that more than 90 percent were contaminated with mold before processing,[7] while another revealed that almost 50 percent of brewed coffees are moldy.[8] Mold is such a problem in coffee that governments around the world—from the European Union to South Korea and Japan—have instituted safe limits for one of the mold toxins in coffee in the parts per billion levels. The United States and Canada, however, have no established limits, resulting in a much higher chance of your cup containing enough mold toxins to influence your performance or even your health. Even the European limits apply to just two types of mold toxins, and they were established for economic reasons, not to maximize human performance. Later in this book you'll see some brand-new, never-before-published research comparing cognitive performance using ultra-low-toxin, lab-tested coffee beans with commonly available commercial beans. The results are astonishing, and provide clear evidence that there is a difference in how your brain works on pure coffee compared to the stuff you probably drink today. Hidden mold toxins in our environment or food, not just those in coffee, impact cognitive performance in everyone.

Clearly, the type of coffee beans you purchase is incredibly important. Cheaper types of coffee cost less because they not only use lower-quality beans, but also include a higher percentage of damaged beans, which are more susceptible to mold toxins. You won't see these mold toxins—they are an invisible by-product of shortcuts coffee producers take when processing green coffee beans. The processing techniques add flavor but unintentionally amplify the amount of toxins in the coffee. Decaf coffee contains more mold on average than caffeinated, partly because coffee people cringe at the thought of ruining high-quality beans with decaf processing and therefore use lower-quality beans to make decaf. It's also because caffeine acts as a natural antifungal defense mechanism that deters mold and other organisms from growing on the beans. When you remove the caffeine, the beans are left defenseless against mold that can form if the beans are stored improperly after roasting.

Even organic and expensive coffees allow mold to grow by using harmful processing methods. When "naturally processed," the beans sit outside, where they collect bird feces and other debris and grow mold. Use of the "wet process" sometimes has better results. With this method, coffee growers toss the beans into giant vats, add water, and let the beans ferment so it's easier to remove the outer parts of the bean. What grows on each batch of the beans is unpredictable, but it usually includes fungal toxins. My research combined with trial-and-error testing taught me how to choose coffee that was more likely to provide the boost without the crash, but the results were not always reliable. I eventually created a process to optimize coffee for brain performance and to verify it with lab testing. Finally, I can drink coffee and feel amazing every time, and tens of thousands of people have experienced a noticeable difference by eliminating just this one daily source of toxin exposure.

Mold toxins aren't found only in coffee; they are commonly found in all sorts of food crops. Mold grows on crops and secretes toxins long before the food is harvested, making this a widespread problem that is not news in the agricultural community. Besides coffee, the main sources of mold toxins in your diet are wheat, corn, and other grains, but peanuts, fruits, chocolate, and wine are often tainted with mold toxins, too. Mold

When I host Champion's Blueprint senior executive development workshops for top business leaders and Fortune 500 CEOs, I always serve Bulletproof Coffee to make sure clients have the highest brain performance and stamina for intense days of leadership development. Bulletproof Coffee always brings amazing clarity and intense focus without hyperactivity to support the highest levels of learning, communication, and awareness. Basically, my events flow better when people's brains are all the way on! **—Dr. Jeff Spencer, leadership author, famed 9-year Tour de France performance coach, Olympic cyclist, and executive performance coach** toxins accumulate in the milk from cows that eat contaminated grains.[9] In fact, products from grain-fed animals often pose a higher mold toxin risk than the grains themselves because the controls on the levels of mold toxins in animal feed are much more lenient than those on grains in the human food supply, and corn-fed and grain-fed animals accumulate mold toxins in their fat. In fact, one of the unacknowledged reasons low-carb diets work is that when you eliminate grains, you end up with a lower level of mold toxins in your food. You are not only what you eat, but also what your food ate!

Mold toxins are sneaky, because there is no way to tell for sure whether or not they are in a certain batch of food. For instance, one bag of nuts maybe perfectly clean, but another bag from a different batch may contain levels of mold toxins that will make you weak—even though you can't taste them. Our big brains make us one of the most susceptible mammals on earth to the effects of mold toxins, and it's important to know that they may be causing your unexplained fatigue or making your focus waiver. This is a common problem among my high-performance clients—and eliminating high-risk foods usually helps with brain focus first. This is why the Bulletproof Diet goes far beyond a regular Paleo or low-toxin diet (Weston A. Price, GAPS [Gut and Psychology Syndrome], etc.) by drastically reducing foods known to be commonly contaminated with mold toxins and acknowledging that they impact how you function long before they make you outright ill.

HACK HUNGER HORMONES

My history of mold exposure provided an opportunity for me to learn more about biohacking than I originally wanted to. When I began biohacking and had my hormone levels tested, I discovered that I had thyroid, adrenal, testosterone, and estrogen problems. I was even diagnosed with Hashimoto's disease, a condition in which the immune system attacks the thyroid gland. In my case, either mold or gluten or both triggered the Hashimoto's, as mold makes your immune system more sensitive to the damaging effects of gluten. I wanted to fix my thyroid, so I began researching the relationship between diet and hormones. I found that saturated fat and cholesterol are the building blocks for all of our hormones, and this is one of the reasons I started experimenting with eating more saturated fat. One of the biggest leaps I took was to begin eating more butter made from the milk of grass-fed cows. This was scary. It went against everything I'd been told about healthy eating my entire life, but I had done the research and checked the science and I wanted to fix my hormones, so I took a deep breath and stopped holding back on butter. I knew that if I was wrong, my body would show more inflammation in blood panels and I could always stop eating it.

Immediately, magical things started to happen. My ability to focus increased, I started losing weight, and my blood panels showed less inflammation, not more—but why? Achieving the desired result didn't satisfy me. As a biohacker, it was important to me to understand the mechanism that had caused it. I continued to research the hormones associated with hunger. Every diet from Atkins to Zone focuses on insulin, the hormone that regulates blood sugar, but I pushed further, trying to determine what controls insulin. This led to a hormone called leptin, which plays an enormous role in weight loss by regulating energy expenditure, appetite, and movement, and it sends a "stop eating!" signal to the brain when you've eaten enough to meet your body's energy demands. It was discovered in 1994, and since then it has unlocked the answers to some of the most confusing aspects of weight loss.

Leptin is produced by fat cells, and your leptin levels are proportionate to your body-fat levels. This means that the fatter you are, the more leptin you have in your body. When you are overweight like I was and have high amounts of circulating leptin in your body for a long period of time, you become leptin resistant. In this case, your brain is constantly bombarded with leptin and doesn't receive the signal that your stomach is full. This leads to sluggishness, weight gain, and the inability to feel satiated.

Leptin resistance is also predictive of insulin resistance, which means that leptin may play a role in controlling insulin sensitivity.[10] Insulin sensitivity itself leads to type 2 diabetes and obesity.

It was clear to me that leptin was a hormone to focus on, but how could I hack it? There are several factors that interfere with leptin sensitivity. As you've read, eating a diet high in foods containing toxic lectin (with a *c*) can contribute to leptin resistance. Also, consuming a lot of fructose also causes leptin resistance by elevating triglyceride levels. Triglycerides impair leptin transport and prevent it from entering the hypothalamus,[11] the structure in the brain that most needs to receive the leptin signal to inhibit hunger.

I designed the Bulletproof Diet to keep triglycerides low by limiting fructose, eliminating food toxins, and reducing food reward and cravings, all of which reset leptin levels and allow for easy weight loss. Sensitizing you to leptin ensures that you only feel hungry when you actually need food, another way that the Bulletproof Diet hacks hunger to keep you focused and energized. Leptin levels drop during short-term fasting and return to normal after eating,[12] making it one reason that Bulletproof Intermittent Fasting (which you'll learn about in detail later) is a painless but important way to retain leptin sensitivity.

When trying to hack a system, hackers instinctively know to look for things that control other things. This kind of thinking led me to research

You guys have saved my life. I was a fat bastard and resigned to an unhealthy life. I tried Bulletproof Coffee because I love coffee, and I automatically started to lose the weight and the food cravings and gain a newfound focus and energy. With this progress, I then started to watch my diet and follow the Bulletproof Diet. I'm now slim, healthy, and loving life. I feel half my age now. You have made an enormous difference to my life. Sincerely, thank you. —**Jose** the amazing symphony of hormones in healthy humans to look for the master control system that manipulates more than just leptin or insulin. It turns out there is another molecule called vasoactive intestinal polypeptide (VIP), which works alongside leptin. VIP is produced by a number of tissues, including the gut, the pancreas, and two important regulatory systems in the brain, the pituitary gland and the hypothalamus. Studies show that when animals don't have enough VIP, their blood sugar, insulin, and leptin all become elevated and the animals crave sweets.[13]

VIP functions as a neuromodulator and neurotransmitter and has many key functions. It can cause changes in the GI tract by modifying hormone and electrolyte levels, modify how the pancreas and gut break down fats and sugars, stimulate bile flow, and control gastric acid release. It can even improve brain function, sleep, and glucose control. In other words, if you don't have healthy VIP levels, you're not going to like how you feel.

VIP is a key modulator of the central nervous system and also has a hand in regulating circadian rhythms, learning and memory, immunity, inflammation, and responses to stress and brain injury.[14] As a biohacker, I knew that if just one hormone controlled so many systems, it was worth paying attention to, and I quickly made regulation of VIP an important focus of the Bulletproof Diet. VIP is crucial for proper brain function and protects against inflammation in the gut. During times of stress, such as when you are exposed to a toxin, VIP production is suppressed. When mice are exposed to toxin from *Aspergillus,* a genus of toxic molds common in food and moldy buildings, VIP levels drop.[15] It's likely that humans experience a drop in VIP when exposed to toxic molds as well.

Since VIP levels are regulated by leptin and vice versa, when leptin isn't working right, VIP also gets thrown out of whack.[16] The Bulletproof Diet sensitizes your body to leptin, which in turn regulates the function of VIP. VIP and leptin are two of the hidden reasons the Bulletproof Diet works so well for so many people. This explains why people feel so good

> The Bulletproof Diet has helped with my overall life and taught me things I will take to the grave—everything from improved mental clarity and motivation to better food and living choices. It has also given me a new way of thinking in the health world, to "hack" my body and brain to make it the best in performance. **—David Reynolds, V8 Supercar driver**

on the Bulletproof Diet, and many often say they feel like a completely new person. They sleep better, think faster, remember more, and live in a state of constant high performance.

MAKE YOUR BODY A DETOXIFICATION MACHINE

Diminishing the inflammation in my body by dramatically reducing toxins and resetting my leptin and VIP levels by eating more healthy fat and less fructose made a huge difference in how I looked and how I felt, but I was still suffering from some strange symptoms. I used to get migraine headaches on occasion, and I had no idea what caused them. They seemed random, but once a migraine hit I'd get sidelined for a few hours at best— hardly the optimal performance I was looking for. Often at the same time, I'd get hives that itched like mad. It seemed likely that something was causing both the headaches and the hives, but I wasn't sure they were related. Like a good biohacker, I tracked my diet and symptoms and researched possible causes until I found out about biogenic amines (BAs).

Biogenic amines are neurotransmitters that influence brain function. Histamine is a BA that is well known for its role in seasonal allergies. When your body makes BAs, they are kept to certain limits, but most people don't realize that BAs like histamine can also be found in certain foods. It's normally no big deal to consume BAs, but they can start to accumulate in your bloodstream if your body fails to detoxify them or if your gut bacteria make extra amines as you digest your food. If your gut bacteria make extra BAs and your liver doesn't have enough enzymes to break them down, your body goes into panic mode to try and get rid of them. It releases adrenaline, increases cardio output and blood sugar levels, and causes higher blood pressure.[17] This leads to inflammation, headaches, and a host of other symptoms you'd never expect.

Histamines and other BAs form when bacteria degrade protein, whether the protein is from vegetables, seeds, or animals like pigs and fish. The single most common source of dietary histamine is fermented soy, particularly soy sauce. I happened to be eating a lot of sushi when I was getting frequent headaches and hives. When I eliminated BAs from my diet, these symptoms disappeared, and I immediately noticed a huge increase in my ability to focus. Many Bulletproof readers have reported fewer seasonal allergies since starting the Bulletproof Diet, and I, too, have experienced a dramatic reduction in the seasonal allergies that used to plague me. This is because the Bulletproof Diet helps modulate the gut bacteria that form histamines while reducing foods that are high in histamines.

HACK YOUR GUT BACTERIA BEFORE THEY HACK YOU

Even after hacking the hives and the migraines, something was still bothering me. The fact that I was so sensitive to BAs told me that my body hadn't been able to detoxify them as well as it should have. That (plus a lifetime of frequent room-clearing gas) meant there was something wrong with my gut bacteria. This really wasn't much of a surprise. As a sickly, overweight kid and young adult, I'd suffered from chronic sinus infections and strep throat for many years and had been on antibiotics about once a month for more than a decade. I knew about the damaging effects of antibiotics, so I'd been eating yogurt for years thinking it would help fix my gut.

Once I realized that wasn't working, I tried everything else I could think of. I bought every expensive probiotic on the planet. Over time I must have spent at least $50,000 on probiotics alone. In 2006, I first tested the species of bacteria in my poo. I even tried helminthic therapy the first year it was discovered. This involved finding a company in Thailand that bred eggs from a parasite called a porcine whipworm, then ordering them and swallowing the eggs so they would hatch in my gut. For some people, this treatment heals the gut by leading to a dramatic reduction in inflammation throughout the body. This may sound pretty radical, and it is, but it's safe because this species of parasite is unable to reproduce in humans and goes away on its own after about 6 weeks. It did not have any effect on me, although it is life changing for some very sick people.

Research on the gut biome taught me why I didn't get the results I wanted from probiotics, especially weight loss. It also helped me understand a vulnerable aspect of my biology that I could use to hack into how my body stored fat. This eventually became a key part of why the Bulletproof Diet works. Studies conducted on mice have provided great insight into how our weight is affected by our gut bacteria rather than just calories in and calories out. When bacteria from the guts of obese mice were placed in the guts of skinny mice, the skinny mice overate by 10 percent and became insulin resistant. When bacteria from lean mice were inserted into the guts of obese mice, they in turn became leaner.[18] Like mice, obese people and lean people have very different gut bacteria. Whether it's the bad gut bacteria that cause obesity or obesity that causes bad gut bacteria is still unknown,[19] but there is evidence that the wrong kind of bacteria in your gut causes insulin resistance and inflammation.[20]

Obese people (and animals) have excess bacteria from the Firmicutes phylum, which includes the *Lactobacillus* bacteria found in yogurt and most probiotic supplements. You need these bacteria, but if they're too active, too plentiful, or from the wrong subtype, you're going to put on fat. Naturally thin people have less Firmicutes and more bacteria from the Bacteroidetes phylum. You can't buy Bacteroidetes species probiotics as a supplement, but you can easily generate them by eating foods that contain their natural food source, which is polyphenols.

Polyphenols are antioxidants that also function as prebiotics for Bacteroidetes. They're found in brightly colored vegetables, but the richest source of polyphenols in Western diets by far is coffee! Chocolate is full of polyphenols, too. Adding more of these superfoods to my diet helped me feed the "thin people" bacteria. This is one hole in the control system that allows the Bulletproof Diet to bend the "calorie rules."

It turns out that gut bacteria—good and bad ones—have already hacked your system. We've become dependent on them in a symbiotic relationship, but that doesn't mean everything they do is in your best interests. This is especially true if you want to be in charge of your fat deposits. Your liver naturally makes a hormone that controls fat storage in a healthy way. Animals without gut bacteria rely on the liver to make that hormone, and they just about never get fat no matter what they eat. Animals with gut bacteria get fatter more easily because gut bacteria *also* make extra fat storage hormones your body doesn't want. Following the Bulletproof Diet allows you to directly hack your gut bacteria in two different ways. First, we make more "thin people" bacteria, and then we manipulate the bacterial fat storage hormones to make them burn fat instead. Welcome to the driver's seat. You'll read more on these techniques in Chapter 4.

Having more good bacteria was a great start, but I wanted to combat the "fat people" bacteria that were hijacking my fat storage systems, too. This led me to the wonders of coconut oil, which is known to be an antifungal agent. Pushing further, I created Brain Octane Oil, a liquid coconut oil extract. Brain Octane Oil is a stronger form of coconut oil with more C8, the most beneficial of the medium-chain triglycerides (MCT), which produces four times the ketones that regular coconut oil does. Interestingly, human breast milk also contains a high percentage of these fats that make the gut a less attractive place for bad bacteria.

Many of the rapid fat-loss benefits of the Bulletproof Diet come from a purposeful change in gut bacteria. This is cutting-edge science, and we'll learn more about this over the next decade. To help in this effort, at my own expense I hosted uBiome at the first-ever Bulletproof Biohacking Conference in San Francisco in January of 2013. uBiome is the first company to set out to allow consumers to measure and understand the genetics of their gut bacteria, and right on their heels came the American Gut Project. This is the far frontier of hacking the human body, and it's all about your poop.

MAKE YOUR BRAIN HAPPY WITH HIGH-PERFORMANCE DETOX SYSTEMS

As I learned more about the role gut bacteria play in detoxing, it made sense to look at the other detox signals in the body. One thing hackers of all kinds do is figure out how to interfere with or take over signaling protocols. If a hacker wanted to prepare a country for invasion, the first thing to do would be to figure out how to take over the communications infrastructure so the left hand wouldn't know what the right hand was doing. I took this approach to signals in the body and looked for signals that control detox mechanisms. Then I could just turn the signal up.

Bile is produced by the liver and passed on to the gallbladder for storage until it's needed for digesting fat; it also acts as a signal for the body to detox. Bile helps break down and absorb fats, so the amount of bile your liver secretes is a factor in weight loss and detoxing. Bile also breaks down toxins for digestion, allowing them to bind to antioxidants and detoxifying agents in your digestive tract. This combination of bile and toxins travels through your GI tract, where much of the bile is reabsorbed while the toxins (hopefully) remain to be excreted. If you don't have enough bile, your body won't be able to bind and excrete enough toxins, and this can lead to an accumulation of toxins in the body.

Consuming fat is a signal for the body to produce more bile, so by eating more healthy fats you can increase bile production and excrete more toxins. This is like changing the oil of your car. Toxins can interfere with bile production, which is yet another reason the Bulletproof Diet is so careful about avoiding them. It's a tricky cycle: The toxins impair bile turnover, and bile turnover is needed to excrete toxins. The Bulletproof Diet hacks this by providing ample amounts of saturated fat, which stimulates the production of bile, and by avoiding toxins that interfere with liver function.

In a relentless pursuit to hack the body to uncover the secrets behind sustained weight loss and peak performance, I ended up creating a science-based diet that goes against everything I'd been told about health and weight loss. How could more butter and less fruit possibly make me feel and look this much better than I ever had before? It turns out that the majority of the dietary wisdom that's been passed down to us is based on a combination of marketing, misinformation, and fear, while medicine naturally tended to focus on isolated things that are easy to measure like total fat or cholesterol. This often means overlooking our bodies' complex systems. But you don't have to rely on advertising or short media articles for information on your health anymore. Thanks to the joys of taking ownership of your own biology, you can directly measure what works for your own biochemistry and what doesn't. Join me in taking back control of your body, your mind, and your performance.

CHAPTER 2

WHAT YOU *THINK* IS GOOD FOR YOU MIGHT BE MAKING YOU FAT, SICK, AND STUPID

After hacking the Bulletproof Diet and discovering how little energy it actually took to lose weight, keep it off, and feel great, I got angry. When I lost my first 50 pounds of fat in 3 months, the number on the scale elated me, but at a deeper level I felt betrayed. I'd struggled for so long to exercise and stick to a low-fat, low-calorie diet, and I felt guilty when it didn't work. Why hadn't my doctors told me about these simple ways to feel better and keep my weight down? Why didn't my parents teach me this? Why weren't people shouting it from the rooftops?

It turns out there are small groups of scientists from different disciplines that have been forming this information, but it can take decades for it to cross over into common knowledge. I made it my mission to meet those scientists, try what they've discovered on myself, and translate that work into useful knowledge that everyone can apply to their own lives. This book is the result of that mission.

There are five basic things your diet should provide: energy for your brain, fuel for your body, nutrients for your cells, no unnecessary toxins, and, perhaps most importantly, satisfaction. But most low-calorie, low-fat diets fail to do *any* of these things. The truth is that many so-called "diet" foods are actually contributing to the obesity epidemic around the world. Let's take a look at some of the diet industry's most commonly perpetuated myths and the Bulletproof take on each of them.

DIET MYTH #1: IF YOU'RE NOT LOSING WEIGHT, YOU'RE NOT TRYING HARD ENOUGH

As a man who grew up fat and used to weigh 300 pounds, this is the myth that caused me the most harm. Trust me, fat people know when we're fat. We are keenly aware of it all the time. We're not lazy—far from it. We spend all day, every day, slowly losing a battle of will against our bodies' biological drive for food. The problem is that dieters and even many doctors woefully misunderstand the concept of willpower. They believe that the secret to success is simply buckling down and saying no to overeating by using an endless reserve of willpower. But willpower has been proven to be a limited resource. You can run out of willpower every day, and it doesn't work to renew your supply simply by deciding to do so.

Decision fatigue is a documented psychological phenomenon that refers to the deteriorating quality of decisions made after a long session of decision

In today's world, we no longer have the luxury of leaving health to chance. Disease is not only predictable but virtually predetermined if one subscribes to a "modern" diet and lifestyle. However, advances in knowledge and science are now revealing the key steps we can all take to ensure a lifetime of vibrant health. Dave Asprey's passion for no-nonsense results is backed by a commitment to thorough research, rigorous testing, and practical application. **—Peter Sage, extreme entrepreneur, endurance athlete, and best-selling author**

The number one reason the Bulletproof Diet is so effective and easy to maintain is that it gives you back your willpower instead of sapping it.

making.[1] For instance, in one study, judges in court were shown to make decisions that were less favorable to defendants later in the day. Decision fatigue may also lead you to make less optimal choices every time you use willpower to choose a "diet" food over one that is more satisfying. The number one reason the Bulletproof Diet is so effective and easy to maintain is that it gives you back your willpower instead of sapping it. It could help you have more energy than you've ever had before by nourishing your cells, balancing your hormone levels, and ending the incessant and exhausting battle with food cravings. The Bulletproof Diet will help you feel satisfied instead of deprived, and when you are satisfied there is no need to waste willpower on something as trivial as food. At first, you will use some willpower to switch from the foods you're accustomed to eating to the better choices, but this won't last long. After just a few days, you'll enjoy making Bulletproof choices because of how amazing they make you feel.

Our bodies have evolved so that our species can survive just about anything the world throws at us, including ice ages, famines, and plagues. You don't need your whole big brain just to eat and reproduce, so different parts of your brain evolved to use different amounts of energy, and your higher-level processes require the most. This means that problems with your energy, whether poor nutrition, toxins, or other stressors, will impact the parts of your brain that use the most energy first. In other words, a process like willpower is far more sensitive to your energy than the lower levels of biology needed for survival.

As new brain imaging techniques reveal the nuances and interconnectedness of different brain structures, it's become obvious that there is no single model or framework that can simplify the brain. I find that the most useful way to think about how the brain uses food is the "triune brain model," which neuroscientist and psychiatrist Paul D. MacLean, MD, developed in the 1960s to explain the brain's structure by dividing it into three parts developed during separate stages of evolution. This model of understanding the brain is debated in the scientific community, but it will help you understand how the Bulletproof Diet hacks the brain so you don't have to waste energy willing yourself not to overeat.

This first part of the brain, which you can think of as your reptile brain, controls low-level processes like temperature regulation and electrical systems. Every creature with vertebrae has a reptile brain, and this brain must get enough nutrients to survive, regardless of what higher parts of the brain need. If you don't get enough energy and nutrients to this part of the brain, you will die. End of story.

All mammals share the second brain—called the limbic brain—which I like to think of as a furry, slobbering "Labrador retriever brain." This one controls the instincts that keep our species alive, like seeking food and reproductive behavior. Your Labrador brain is only trying to help you survive, but it ends up working against you in three main ways. The first is that it is distractible. Like a dog, we're always looking around for potential sticks to chase instead of focusing on what's right in front of us. Having a hard time paying attention? That's your Labrador brain triggering your fight-or-flight response to make sure you're safe. The second way your Labrador brain works against you is also related to species survival, this time to support reproduction. Your Labrador brain distracts you with inappropriate urges and makes sure you spend a lot of time and energy trying to satisfy them. (At least that part is enjoyable!) The final way our Labrador brains get us in trouble is a main focus of this book—they make us want to eat anything and everything we can get our paws on. Your Labrador brain wants you to eat things indiscriminately to make sure you don't die of starvation.

When you eat a food that contains things that are harmful to your system, it can trigger a fight-or-flight response—one that can be measured as your heart rate—along with a strong craving for sugary foods that will provide a quick burst of energy to deal with the threat. You experience this as a food craving, which I define as a strong need to eat that goes beyond simple hunger. Unfortunately, many people experience food cravings so often that they've forgotten what hunger without a simultaneous craving feels like.

When you resist the craving, you are using your third and final brain, which MacLean called the neocortex and I like to call the "human brain." Remember, the reptile brain is first in line to get the nutrients and calories it needs, followed by your Labrador brain, so your human brain gets the leftovers. If you only eat enough food to keep the first two brains happy or eat the wrong things, your human brain runs out of energy first, which means you run out of willpower. The next thing you know, you give in to your craving and wake up halfway through a pint of ice cream.

Traditional weight-loss diets don't provide enough fuel for all three brains. When you go on one of these diets, every time you see food, your Labrador says, "You're starving! Survival is at stake! Eat that NOW!" You're then forced to use your willpower to say, "No! Bad dog!" This happens again and again until you begin suffering from decision-making fatigue and your supply of willpower runs out, often by the middle of the day.

For example, if you eat a low-fat, low-calorie breakfast your body will secrete insulin, which allows your cells to use the sugar you just ingested and thus causes your blood sugar level to drop. Your Labrador will start to panic because it thinks the body is running out of the fuel it needs to stay alive. The Labrador starts to pester you to eat something sweet to raise your blood sugar. This is how your biology evolved to keep you from starving to death, but it's not serving you any longer. What your body perceived as an emergency was just you following your diet! By the time lunch comes around, you're completely out of willpower and you give in and eat pizza or fried chicken or fast food. Or maybe you try to bribe the Labrador by eating just one piece of candy with your fat-free lunch. Does this sound familiar?

Another common scenario is that you eat a big breakfast that contains either toxins or foods that you're sensitive to. Eating a food you're sensitive to can trigger your fight-or-flight response, and your Labrador demands sugar to give you enough extra energy to run away. If the food contains toxins, your liver uses blood sugar to oxidize the toxins, which causes a drop in available energy for your brain. The result is that you feel like you need sugar right away.

To use your diet to manipulate your brain, you have to know which foods tell your Labrador brain that you're starving by either causing a drop in blood sugar or stimulating a fight-or-flight response. On the Bulletproof Diet, foods are broken down into three categories, which we'll discuss in further detail later. There are Bulletproof foods that you can almost always eat freely, Suspect foods to approach with caution because they might cause a craving for you, and Kryptonite foods that almost always limit your performance, make you weak, and should be avoided altogether.

While some foods like high-fructose corn syrup are Kryptonite for everyone, each of us also has some foods that are our own personal Kryptonite. For example, chocolate is a healthy Bulletproof food for most people, but for someone who is sensitive to it, chocolate is Kryptonite. Most people are blissfully unaware that some foods they eat all the time are secretly making them weak and causing cravings. By getting a food allergy blood test, you'll learn which Suspect foods are guilty of wrecking your performance. This will help you to become truly Bulletproof.

DIET MYTH #2: YOU'RE NOT AS HUNGRY AS YOU THINK YOU ARE

Hunger decreases your performance, saps your energy, and makes you cranky, tired, and unproductive. It also decreases your willpower by activating your Labrador brain. Sustained hunger is not a sign of toughness or resolve, and it's definitely not Bulletproof. Ironically, when I weighed 300 pounds, I was hungry all the time, and I was less productive than I am now because I was thinking about food all day long. Back when I was an arrogant young millionaire, I'd end meetings early, before lunchtime, by saying, "I have to eat now so our meeting is over, sorry about that." Then, I'd go eat a lunch that left me with even more cravings. I didn't mean to sound like a jerk. My hunger just got the best of me. My Labrador brain was winning.

Let's face it: Being hungry is a massive waste of time. It takes your attention away from more important matters and increases the number of mistakes you make on any given task. It also saps your willpower and drive. When you're hungry, you're far more likely to go home and watch TV instead of working for an extra hour on your business plan. If you added up all the hours that most dieters waste either thinking about their hunger or abandoning tasks because they can't focus, it would probably come to at least several hours a day. Imagine how much more you could achieve in 1 week if you had a few extra hours each day, and how much nicer you'd be to others if you weren't so hungry!

In its simplest form, hunger is the urge to eat. It's an instinct that keeps humans from starving to death—part of our Labrador brains. The goal of a diet shouldn't be to ignore hunger or to sate it by eating a low-calorie snack every 90 minutes. Instead, the Bulletproof Diet hacks hunger by balancing the hormones that control this instinct. The biochemistry of hunger is complex and driven by hormones produced throughout the body. It's primarily two opposing hormones that are in the driver's seat of your hunger. Ghrelin, which is produced by cells in the stomach's lining, turns on hunger and turns off satiety. Leptin, as I already mentioned, turns off hunger by turning on satiety and is produced by fat cells. When your small intestine detects protein in the food you've eaten, it helps leptin stimulate satiety, and when the pancreas detects fat in your intestines, it releases a hormone that prevents ghrelin from turning off the satiety call. On the flip side, fructose, the primary sugar in fruit, does a worse job of turning off the hunger-hormone ghrelin than almost any other food.

Feeling intense hunger or "I need to eat now or I'm going to crash" is a sign that whatever you ate earlier in the day wasn't actually satiating because it didn't turn off ghrelin and/or turn on leptin. On the other hand, feeling a mild, "I ought to eat something in the next couple of hours" hunger doesn't weaken your performance and is easy to handle. Because your hunger hormones will be well managed on the Bulletproof Diet, that's the only type of hunger you'll ever feel.

It's time to get back those hours you wasted feeling hungry and make good use of them. By eating foods with high-quality fats and plenty of calories, the Bulletproof Diet will allow you to avoid the performance-robbing, brain-sapping problem called hunger while losing weight more quickly and effortlessly than ever before. Hunger isn't something to ignore, but it is extremely controllable. You are not weak if you give in to your food cravings. You are simply eating the wrong things or not enough of the right things! By following the Bulletproof Diet, you'll take control of your biology so that hunger is no longer a distraction.

DIET MYTH #3: A LOW-FAT DIET IS HEALTHY

In the 1950s, a scientist named Ancel Keys rocked the world of nutrition by claiming, with some pretty convincing research, that saturated fat caused heart disease. The low-fat diet craze immediately stormed the scene and has unfortunately stuck around ever since, despite the fact that we later learned Keys threw out data that didn't fit his model.[2] In other words, he manipulated the research to make it look like it backed his theory that saturated fat caused heart disease, but in fact the science didn't support his theory at all.

Food chemists immediately began concocting low-fat foods. When removing the fat from these foods, they had to replace it with something. The two choices were sugar or protein. Well, sugar tastes better than protein and is more affordable, so excessive sugar or corn syrup were pumped into most low-fat "diet" foods. These low-fat foods are actually terrible for you because they not only lack nutrients and replace satiating fats with sugar and starch, but they also taste like cardboard and make your Labrador brain believe a famine is coming.

Dietary fat contains more energy per gram than any other nutrient, so it is most effective at delivering energy to the parts of your body that need it. Compared to protein or sugar, fat also has the least impact on insulin levels. Low-fat foods containing sugar spike insulin, which leads to energy crashes and weight gain. Fat also doesn't raise the stress hormone cortisol, which increases blood sugar and suppresses your immune system, as much as protein or carbohydrates.

One of the main reasons people fail on so many diets is that they feel like they're being tortured and simply give up and go back to eating the foods they actually enjoy. But the truth is that you can lose weight by enjoying delicious, satiating foods on the Bulletproof Diet. And you can eat as much as your Labrador brain wants as long as you're eating the right foods. When you eat real foods that aren't designed with flavor-enhancing chemicals that trick you into eating more, your Labrador brain tells you to stop eating when you've had enough. You won't want more food than your body needs.

Fat is the foundation of the Bulletproof Diet, but not all fats are created equal. Later in the book, you'll learn which types of fats turn off cravings and which types cause them. Unfortunately, when low-fat foods became popular, we started rejecting all fats instead of just the bad ones. This type of thinking has stuck around for far too long. Rather than experiencing more of the same fat-free agony, now you can reap the health benefits of a high-healthy-fat diet and wake up every morning thrilled about the food you're going to eat that day. The most effective diet in the world won't work if you don't stick with it. One simple reason the Bulletproof Diet is so effective over the long term is that it tastes good and doesn't cause your Labrador brain to waste your willpower battling cravings. This makes it sustainable. Why would you ever go off a diet that tastes better than the diet you were eating before you started looking great, losing weight, and kicking ass?

DIET MYTH #4: EATING FAT WILL MAKE YOU FAT

Thanks to Ancel Keys, we're not only stuck with unhealthy fat-free foods, but also have grown afraid of eating fat because we believe it will make us fat and sick. In fact, the idea that eating fat will make you fat is nothing more than a myth. As I was creating and testing the Bulletproof Diet, I wanted to see how quickly eating more fat calories would make me fat. I figured that if what we've been taught about diets is true, I'd gain a pound of fat for every extra 3,500 calories I ate, especially if I ate tons of fat. To really stack the deck against myself for the experiment, on August 6, 2009, I stopped exercising, cut my sleep to less than 5 hours a night (which is also supposed to make you fat), and started eating between 4,000 and 4,500 calories from the Bulletproof Diet each day. About 70 percent of those calories came from Bulletproof fats.

According to most nutritionists, I should have gained a dozen pounds in a month of eating this way. Instead, the opposite happened. Suddenly, I was on fire. My brain worked effortlessly, I didn't need more sleep, and I even grew a six-pack. I couldn't believe it, and I'll admit that I spent a lot of time in front of the mirror marveling at how flat my stomach was becoming as I literally stuffed myself with food.

I didn't want to stop the experiment because life felt just grand, so I ended up doing it for 2 years straight. I used my extra energy to launch the Bulletproof Executive blog while gaining accolades for my full-time work as a vice president at a big technology company. The calorie counters predicted that after 2 years I should have weighed 600 pounds, but the only weight I actually gained was a few pounds of muscle. I finally backed off on the calories because it's a lot of work (not to mention expensive) to eat that much. It's also not necessary or even advisable.

Thanks to faulty research, fats have gained a bad reputation, but the right types of fats are healthy and essential for life. All nutrients are converted inside the body before being used. The right fats are clean-burning, nutritious, and satisfying energy sources that keep your body and brain functioning at maximum capacity. Fat is a building block of healthy cell walls and hormones and is needed for fertility, temperature regulation, and shock absorption. Some vitamins—A, E, D, and K—are fat soluble, meaning that they need fat in order to be absorbed in the body.

To put it simply, healthy fats are an important component of the human body. It's what we're made of. The healthy female body is about 29 percent fat, while men are about 15 percent fat. Portions of every part of our bodies

> This diet has allowed me to feel, look, and be better than I ever have been before. Because of that, I want to share this information with everyone that wants to listen and wake up! I am a true believer and advocate. It is time to unlearn, folks! **—Davis**

are made of fat, including our brains. This means that low-fat diets starve our brains. Our brains and our bodies need some "essential" fats, like omega-3s, to function, but our bodies cannot produce them. We have to consume these fats in our diet in the correct ratios and amounts. While many people have become downright afraid of fat, eating the right kinds does not promote weight gain or pose any type of health risk at all. Because the healthy fats in the Bulletproof Diet help maintain and balance the hormone levels in your body, the result is weight loss rather than weight gain.

DIET MYTH #5: CUTTING CALORIES IS THE BEST WAY TO LOSE WEIGHT

Maybe you're thinking that if it's not fat that makes you fat, then consuming a lot of calories must be the culprit. Indeed, many diets claim that the magic formula to weight loss is "fewer calories in than calories out." This is sort of true in a famine situation—it *is* possible to starve yourself thin, at least for a little while, and if you lock someone in a metabolic chamber in a lab, you can achieve a true caloric deficit by measuring their actual caloric output and providing food accordingly. But we now know that crash diets mess with your hunger hormones and your metabolism, making it easier for you to gain weight later when you begin eating normally again. Insulin resistance, leptin resistance, low testosterone, and thyroid problems are all potential consequences of low-calorie diets.

Regardless of calories, a diet's number one purpose should be to fuel and nourish your mind and body. Did you know that your brain actually uses up to 25 percent of your daily calories? With that in mind, is it any surprise that you feel tired and lose motivation if you exercise more and cut calories to lose weight? Your Labrador brain takes all the calories, and your human brain is left running on fumes.

I'm not saying that calories don't matter—quite the opposite. In order to feel in control of your biology, it's essential to eat enough calories. Your Labrador brain responds to the stress of restricted calories and intense workouts the same way it would to a famine or other natural disaster—by conserving energy. This leads to brain fog, fatigue, weight gain, and a broken thyroid. It also leaves you feeling hungry all the time.

Besides the fact that cutting calories too much does not help you lose more weight, the formula "fewer calories in than calories out" has some pretty big loopholes—ones biohackers can take advantage of! In the animal ranching industry, there is a measure called "feed efficiency." By giving estrogen to cattle, the cattle can get fat on 30 percent fewer calories. This saves a lot of money for the ranchers, and leaves you eating beef with added estrogen that might make you fat just like it did the cattle. So if a tiny dose of a hormone can make a cow fat on 30 percent less calories, clearly the number of calories you eat isn't the only factor determining whether you'll gain or lose weight.

It's also important to know that up to 50 percent of your individual calorie burn is related to things that can't easily be tracked, such as room temperature, sleep, altitude, and how hard you breathe. So for most people, there's no accurate way to deduce the number of calories used daily or even whether those are fat calories or sugar calories. It's also important to take into account the fact that different foods do different things to your body. This is a simple and seemingly obvious concept that goes against what most diets tell you. But think about it this way—if a calorie was just a calorie, you'd be able to lose weight eating just high-fructose corn syrup or a bottle of canola oil. What we've found instead is that over time these foods destroy your body, your brain, and your performance, and they don't necessarily lead to weight loss even if you're technically consuming fewer calories.

When you start focusing not on the number of calories you consume but rather the quality of your food and the nutrition it provides, your body will respond in kind, revving up its fat-burning and nutrient absorption and naturally regulating your caloric intake. This results in the weight loss and mental clarity that so many people are already experiencing on the Bulletproof Diet.

DIET MYTH #6: EVERYTHING NATURAL IS GOOD FOR YOU

How many times have you been told to "eat more fruits and vegetables"? It's almost as if "fruits and vegetables" has become a single word. The only problem is that from a nutritional perspective, fruits and vegetables have as much in common as fish and bicycles. People like to tout the health benefits of fruits by calling them "nature's candy," but the truth is that fruits actually have more in common with candy than they do with vegetables. Fruits are primarily made of sugar and water with a bit of fiber, while vegetables are low in sugar and extremely high in nutrients.

The biggest problem with fruits is the main sugar they contain, fructose. As I already mentioned when discussing leptin, your liver converts fructose to either glucose or triglycerides, the latter of which are then stored as fat. And fructose not only causes you to gain fat through these biochemical pathways, but also doesn't suppress your appetite after you eat it the way protein or fats do. Fructose isn't even as satiating as other sugar sources, so you're more likely to overconsume it[3] than any other type of sugar. There are few faster ways to cause a food craving than to eat or drink something with a lot of fructose like dried fruit, fruit juice, soda, or even a piece of whole fruit.

Eating fructose isn't just bad for your waistline; it can contribute to heart disease and damaged arteries in a number of ways. The first, as I mentioned, is by elevating triglycerides, a well-established predictor of heart disease. Fructose also easily links to proteins such as collagen, the main connective tissue in the skin and arteries, and to fats. When linking to collagen, fructose creates toxic advanced glycation end products, or AGEs for short. ("Glycation" refers to the linking of sugar molecules with proteins, DNA, and fats.) These are aptly named, as these end products play a role in the aging process and create additional oxidative stress in the body.[4] AGEs not only are a major cause of skin wrinkles, but also age arteries and can lead to atherosclerosis.

Fructose is also damaging to the body because it feeds the bad bacteria in your gut. When fructose enters the gut, disease-causing bacteria preferentially eat it and reproduce. This is likely one of the reasons there is an epidemic of small intestinal bacterial overgrowth (SIBO).[5] Some of the bad bacteria that love fructose create uric acid as a by-product of their own metabolism. When too much uric acid builds up in the body, it can lead to deposits of sharp uric acid crystals in the joints, under the skin, and even in the kidneys, where they cause kidney stones. When you have these uric acid deposits throughout the body, you have gout, one of the most painful and debilitating forms of arthritis. A disturbing number of my friends and colleagues in Silicon Valley have dealt with gout as early as in their 30s. Their doctors have told them it's due to meat consumption, but I've been counseling these friends for a decade to reduce their fructose intake to help get rid of their gout. This has been more successful than reducing the amount of meat they eat, although the Bulletproof Diet is a moderate-protein diet, not a high-protein one.

In mainstream medicine, the health benefits of fruits are overstated while the health risks of fructose are completely ignored, but there are some doctors out there who have begun warning about the dangers of fructose. Robert Lustig, MD, a leading health expert, the author of *Fat Chance,* and a specialist in pediatric endocrine disorders at the University of California, San Francisco, has come to the conclusion that even "average" levels of fructose can inhibit performance in a major way. Eating anything more than a little bit of fructose daily is simply not good for your brain or your body, and that's why the Bulletproof Diet limits fructose to *no more than* 25 grams a day and preferably less. That's roughly the amount in 2 large apples. My 100 excess pounds of fat wouldn't budge when I was eating several pieces of fruit a day, and now I understand why! Avoiding excessive fructose is one of the best things you can do to slim your waistline and absolutely decimate food cravings. So much for "An apple a day keeps the doctor away." Instead, the saying should be, "Three apples a day keeps the doctor well paid."

DIET MYTH #7: YOU HAVE TO WORK OUT A LOT TO LOSE WEIGHT

When I weighed 300 pounds, I spent a lot of time and energy in the gym trying to lose weight. What an enormous waste! Thanks to the joys of biohacking, self-experimenting, and working with world-class experts, now I don't have to spend nearly as much time on my physique to stay lean and muscular. I eat tons of fat and don't ever have to worry about burning it off because my body efficiently metabolizes fat for energy. Thanks to the hacks I used to develop the Bulletproof Diet and Bulletproof Intermittent Fasting (which I'll discuss in detail later), my body easily switches from burning sugar to burning fat for energy.

One of the greatest misconceptions when it comes to weight loss is that burning calories is relevant to losing pounds and slimming down. That's because your diet is much more important than exercise when it comes to weight loss. But perhaps the most earth-shattering thing I've discovered about exercise through biohacking is that overtraining can actually cause you to gain weight. That's right—working out too much can actually backfire against your weight-loss goals. If you're exercising every day to lose weight, you might be stacking the deck against yourself!

Your body responds to rigorous exercise as it does to any other stressor: by increasing cortisol levels in your body. Cortisol is a hormone that increases blood sugar, suppresses the immune system, and even decreases bone formation. When cortisol levels remain raised for extended periods of time, the well-known result is weight gain and muscle loss. This is not to say that movement and exercise are forbidden on the Bulletproof Diet. Moving around is great for your nervous system, brain, and detox systems. I enjoy being active and recommend a Bulletproof workout regimen later in the book so that you can do a small amount of rigorous exercise once a week in order to get the benefits many people seek from daily workouts. But working out is not necessary for weight loss on the Bulletproof Diet. It's the foods you eat that will help you lose weight, build muscle, and stay in the best shape of your life.

DIET MYTH #8: COFFEE IS BAD FOR YOU

You've already read about the negative health effects of mold toxins that are unfortunately extremely common in coffee. But many people still believe that coffee itself, even without mold, is bad for you. Coffee has been the target of ruthless misinformation campaigns from companies selling coffee substitutes for almost 100 years. In fact, many of the negative things you may believe about coffee likely came from ad campaigns from the 1920s. At the time, the company that now makes Post Cereal sold a burnt-grain coffee substitute called Postum by claiming it was healthier than coffee, a myth that still persists even if Postum has been relegated to a fringe food product.

The studies on coffee and health go back and forth. Some studies show health benefits while others show negative impacts. This might seem confusing, but the reason is simple: Bad coffee is bad for you, and scientists don't differentiate between *types* of coffee when they run these studies. They don't control for processing methods or the source of the beans, and the vast majority of studies use instant coffee from the grocery store, which is shown to be higher in mold toxins than brewed coffee, or depend on participants self-reporting coffee consumption, so there is no control over the quality of the beverage. In short, the studies that show negative effects from drinking coffee—and there are some—never controlled for the presence of mold toxins in the coffee. The mold toxins themselves could explain many of the negative coffee studies.

When you eliminate the effects of mold and look at the whole picture, it's clear that coffee is more of a "superfood" than anything else in your diet. In study after study, coffee—even with mold—has been shown to improve focus, memory recall, and performance. Other studies show it lowers the risk of stroke and diabetes.[6] As I mentioned in Chapter 1, it provides large amounts of polyphenols that feed good bacteria in the gut.[7] Red wine and chocolate are famous for their polyphenol content, but coffee actually has far greater quantities. The Fred Hutchinson Cancer Research Center discovered that men who drank four or more cups of coffee per day had a 59 percent lower chance of prostate cancer recurrence. Coffee also has powerful thermogenic properties, meaning that it stimulates fat loss and even helps build muscle (when used properly) by repressing a substance in your body called mTOR, which I'll discuss in detail later. Coffee is also a powerful antioxidant. In fact, it's the number one source of dietary antioxidants in the US diet. It is even being studied for anticancer use.[8]

When you mix low-toxin coffee with the right fats, you get an amazing drink that stomps on hunger and cravings, lights up your brain with an alternative energy source, and helps you lose weight, build muscle, and increase focus and performance without the negative effects of moldy coffee. This drink, Bulletproof Coffee, is a core part of the diet, and I can't wait for you to try it.

DIET MYTH #9: SALT IS A HAZARDOUS SUBSTANCE

In 1979, when I was 7 years old, the US Surgeon General stated, "Unequivocally, studies . . . show a cause-effect relationship between high salt intake and elevated blood pressure." Because of this, I always felt morally superior when I restricted my sodium, but the problem is that human beings cannot live without salt. Having the right amount of it in your body is essential. Plus, your body needs a lot more salt when you're stressed because salt is an important part of your adrenal response. As you probably know, your adrenal glands produce many of your hormones, including the stress hormone cortisol. When you are chronically stressed and your adrenals continue making high levels of cortisol, the adrenals become fatigued and cannot produce other important hormones. One of these hormones is aldosterone, which balances sodium and potassium levels in the body. When the adrenals are too stressed to secrete aldosterone, you can become dehydrated and have low blood pressure, and as a result you often crave salt. I learned this the hard way when I went through a period of extreme adrenal burnout. The test results below show my norepinephrine to epinephrine level at a score of 46. Anything over 8 means extreme adrenal fatigue.

To bring myself back to a state of resilience and health, I had to add a lot more salt to my diet. Since then, I've been increasing my energy throughout the day by taking ½ to 1 teaspoon of sea salt in water right when I wake up. That's when your body uses salt the most efficiently.

Much has been made of the supposed negative health effects of salt, but the science shows that low-sodium diets are actually the ones that cause harm. According to a summary of 23 studies printed in the *American Journal of Hypertension,* restricting sodium to less than 2,500 milligrams per day not only causes aldosterone to become deregulated as I just explained, but it also makes your plasma renin activity go up, which increases your risk

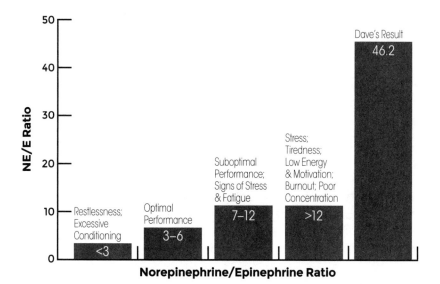

of heart attack dramatically. In addition, your insulin resistance increases, which makes you fat. Your sympathetic nerve activity—your fight-or-flight response—goes up. Your serum cholesterol goes up. And your triglyceride levels go up, too.[9]

The maximum level of sodium currently recommended by experts is 2,300 milligrams, but this research concluded that the right level of sodium for most people is between 2,500 and 6,000 milligrams per day and that the constant push to lower sodium in people's diets is increasing their stress and potentially causing heart attacks. Another study shows that an increase in dietary sodium may decrease plasma apolipoprotein B.[10] This lipoprotein is associated with coronary heart disease even more than LDL.[11] While many doctors claim that salt intake leads to high blood pressure, studies show that only certain people who already have high blood pressure react this way to salt.[12] High blood pressure can actually be caused by many factors, including too little calcium, magnesium, or potassium.

Many people think of sodium and salt as synonymous, but they are not actually the same thing. The stuff that we commonly call "table salt" is actually a mix of chemically extracted pure sodium and toxic aluminum anticaking agents. Consuming these fillers can lead to excess sodium in the blood, which causes problems like rheumatism, arthritis, gout, kidney stones, and gallstones. High-quality sea salt, however, provides the sodium the body needs and helps maintain mineral balance without the toxic aluminum agents. The best salt I've found is pink salt mined in Utah or the Himalayas from pollutant-free ancient seabeds. But switching from table salt to any kind of sea salt will give you a massive upgrade, while including more salt in your diet will help you combat stress while feeling strong and powerful.

DIET MYTH #10: MODERATION IS THE KEY TO SUCCESS WHEN DIETING

Conventional wisdom tells us, "Everything in moderation," but in this case conventional wisdom is just plain wrong. There is no argument for lead or cyanide "in moderation," and when you want to perform at your peak it's a terrible idea to consume even moderate amounts of toxins that will make you tired, give you brain fog, and crush your performance a few hours later. It's important to know that every little thing you put in your mouth affects your performance in some way or another. Some toxins can make you stronger, but others, like mold toxins that damage DNA, have no positive benefits at any dose.

The Bulletproof Diet is not an all-or-nothing approach; it's a simple roadmap that will help you make better choices so you can eat more of the foods that move your health and performance in the right direction and fewer of the ones that don't support your goals. If you do choose to eat some nutritional Kryptonite, you're not a bad person, and you haven't fallen off the wagon. Perhaps your Labrador brain got the best of you, or maybe you made a conscious decision to eat a food you dearly love even though you know it won't help your performance. But if you're unaware of which foods will make you Bulletproof and which ones will act as Kryptonite even in small quantities, you're helpless in this decision. This goes for foods that are Kryptonite for everyone, like gluten, soy, and MSG (monosodium glutamate), and Suspect foods that are Bulletproof for some people and Kryptonite for others. Sprouted gluten-free grains might be neutral for some people, but if you're sensitive to them, they're Kryptonite for you. You're the one who counts!

By using the 2-Week Protocol later in the book, you'll learn how to tell which foods make you feel Bulletproof and will finally be fully in charge of your body. This will hand you the keys to feeling great, looking good, and mastering your demanding life. "Everything in moderation" leads to just moderate performance. Reject moderation and aim for something greater. Moderation has nothing to do with being Bulletproof.

CHAPTER

3

STOP COUNTING CALORIES, EAT MORE FAT, AND TRUST YOUR HUNGER

Long conversations with antiaging experts and biochemists at the Silicon Valley Health Institute (SVHI) combined with my own research and biohacking revealed some basic principles that were counterintuitive and flipped what I thought I knew about dieting on its head. As a leader of SVHI, I had the chance to learn from a bevy of medical and nutrition experts who taught me that nutrition is far more complex than just counting calories. They showed me that our simple models for thinking about food don't work no matter how much we want them to or how easy they are to talk about. Despite what I saw everywhere in the press, eating more of the right fats and calories seemed to be the secret to gaining shocking amounts of power and energy, feeling awesome, getting my brain back online, and losing weight so easily that it almost felt accidental.

As I dug deeper to find out which sources of fats and calories would give me the absolute best, most consistent results, the Bulletproof Diet began to take shape. I discovered that fat isn't good or bad. Protein isn't good or bad. Even carbs aren't good or bad. Food and macronutrients are more complex than that, but the hacks I developed will make it seem simple.

FANTASTIC FATS

Fat is the most important and least inflammatory macronutrient, and on the Bulletproof Diet, 50 to 70 percent of your daily calories should come from the right kinds of fats. This is not a license to eat whatever kinds of fat you find! There are some "bad" fats that really will make you fat, but eating significant amounts of the right types of fat will not. In fact, when you eat more healthy fats, your body becomes better equipped to naturally turn it into energy. We're often told to avoid fat because it has more calories, but when we build a high-performance car to go faster, we design it to use high-octane fuel, which stores more energy per gallon than low-octane fuel. We measure the octane of food using calories, and when you teach your body to burn fat for energy it becomes a higher-performance machine, complete with a kind of energy that's normally unavailable.

Our cells, organs, and brains are all made of fat and need high-quality fat to function optimally. Fat is also the basis for the lining of your nerves, called myelin, which allows electricity to flow efficiently. When you have more myelin, you literally think faster. When people hear that they should eat more fat, they often start to worry about cholesterol, but cholesterol is so vital that your liver manufactures it according to your body's needs! Cholesterol isn't necessarily an enemy. Even if you managed to consume no cholesterol through your diet, your body would still produce the amount of cholesterol it requires for many basic functions. Fat-containing cholesterol helps build the outer coating of your cells, makes up the bile acids that you need to digest foods in your intestines, and provides the building blocks for your hormones and vitamin D.

When you eat enough of the right fats without excess carbs, your body

> Getting most of my calories from healthy fats (especially high-quality saturated fats) has made a huge difference in my satiation, energy, and physical performance. As a competitive obstacle course racer and rock climber, such a diet has allowed me to perform and recover optimally while logging very minimal training hours. I am eager to continue self-experimenting and learning more Bulletproof strategies for optimal performance. —**Andrew Thomas, nutritionist**

learns to efficiently burn fat for fuel and to form healthy cell membranes. This is because your body burns carbs first. On average, men should aim for at least 120 to 150 grams of fat (8 to 10 tablespoons) per day. Women should aim for at least 90 to 120 grams (6 to 8 tablespoons) per day, although your body weight, activity level, genetics, and hunger all play roles in determining the exact right amount for you. That's why I recommend that healthy fats make up a range between 50 and 70 percent of the calories you eat each day.

So, what are the "right" kinds of fat? Nutritionist and early trans fats researcher Mary Enig, PhD, has long been a proponent of a diet high in healthy fats. She developed two basic ways to understand fats. The first is to look at how long a fat molecule is. As a general rule for edible fats, the shorter the fat, the rarer and more anti-inflammatory it is. This is why the Bulletproof Diet ensures that you get adequate amounts of the harder-to-find short- and medium-chain fats, which include the butyric acid found in butter and several types of medium-chain triglycerides found in coconut oil.

The second way to understand your fat is to see how stable it is. Oxygen is vital for life, but it also drives very strong chemical reactions like rusting and oxidation and is responsible for damaging fats. The most stable fats are saturated because saturated fat molecules have fewer places for oxygen to damage them through oxidation. Oxidized (damaged) fats cause you to age more quickly, create inflammation in the body, and make less-effective cell membranes. When your body has no choice but to incorporate oxidized fats into cell membranes, the damaged fats create free radicals and put a burden on your system. This is why your body uses saturated fats to make cell membranes and hormones. The second most stable fat is monounsaturated fat, which is relatively stable because there is only one place where oxygen can damage it ("mono" = one).

Unsaturated fats are the least stable and most inflammatory fats, but our bodies do need some of them, such as omega-3s and omega-6s, two different kinds of unsaturated fats. Omega-3 and omega-6 fats have unique chemical structures and do different things in the body. In particular, omega-3s have anti-inflammatory benefits and are more difficult to find in standard Western diets, since most refined vegetable oils (which I'll discuss in detail later) consist of polyunsaturated omega-6s. Poultry, the most common protein in Western diets, is also high in omega-6s. For this reason, the Bulletproof Diet focuses on increasing your intake of omega-3s from sources like fish and krill oil and reducing (but not entirely eliminating) omega-6s. It's important to have the right balance of omega-3s and omega-6s.

As you read in the previous chapter, saturated fats have been vilified ever since Ancel Keys used faulty research to back his claim that they lead to heart disease, but an exhaustive analysis of 76 academic studies involving more than 600,000 participants found that saturated fat consumption is in fact **not** associated with coronary disease risk.[1] This is well known in the antiaging world where I cut my teeth, and it's baked into (pun intended) the Bulletproof Diet.

PREFERRED PROTEINS

I spent years on a high-protein diet with limited saturated fats and lots of monounsaturated fats, and I experienced the same problems I often see in my clients on low-carb diets. They lose a great deal of weight by increasing protein and reducing carbohydrates, but their weight loss stalls before they reach their ideal weight, and brain fog often sets in. I lost 50 pounds of fat and inflammation in 3 months using a high-protein diet, but the other 50 pounds I wanted to lose wouldn't budge, and it was taking a lot of willpower to keep the first 50 off. After years of experimenting, I even tried a raw vegan diet that was very low in protein out of desperation. For a little while, it worked really well, and I noticed a dramatic decrease in my overall levels of inflammation. I realized that my previous diets had included too much protein, which was contributing to inflammation. But after a few months as a raw vegan, I noticed that my health was not moving in the right direction, so I added more protein to my diet, but this time in moderate amounts, and I focused on quality protein. That's when I really started to thrive. Had I not cut protein out of my diet to such an extent, I probably wouldn't have realized that too much protein had been causing inflammation. When I did the research, I learned that scientists have indeed found that excess protein can cause inflammation because it is more difficult for the body to digest than other macronutrients.

Compared to healthy fats, protein itself is metabolically difficult to turn into glucose for energy. This is because your liver requires a source of fuel to efficiently process protein, and that fuel must come from either fat or glucose. This is one reason a low-fat, zero-added-sugar, and high-protein meal can leave you feeling full but still cause you to crave sweets later in the day. Without a good source of glycogen or fat, your body needs sugar to digest all that protein. Over the last 30 years, high-protein diets have become synonymous with health because these diets are often low in sugar and fat. But the truth is that while a high-protein, low-fat diet is superior to a high-carbohydrate diet, you'll get the very best results from a diet with moderate amounts of protein and ample healthy fats, too.

The Bulletproof Diet focuses on adequate (but not excessive) amounts

The Bulletproof Diet has made the biggest impact on my brain fog. Eating this way gives me the focus and willpower to be in the zone at the tables for as long as it takes to win! —**Nam Le, world poker champion** of very-high-quality protein. Just as different fats affect your body differently, the type of protein you eat has a unique impact on your immune system, inflammation, and muscle gain. The oversimplified idea that "protein is healthy" has allowed the processed-food industry to stuff their products with low-quality proteins, including gluten and soy. (I'll talk about these Kryptonite foods in more detail later.) By focusing on less-inflammatory, more-bioavailable proteins that your body can easily process on the Bulletproof Diet, you'll have higher-quality raw materials for your body and get more energy than you would from eating larger amounts of lower-quality proteins.

Of course, if you're a high-performance athlete or trying to gain a lot of muscle, you should consume more protein than the average person to support that goal. But for most people, up to 20 percent of your daily calories should come from Bulletproof protein sources such as low-mercury fish, grass-fed beef and lamb, pastured eggs, hydrolyzed collagen, gelatin, and clean whey concentrate. Poultry is a somewhat inferior protein that should be eaten in moderation. Protein is so important to your survival for maintaining muscle mass and bone density that your body and brain have powerful feedback mechanisms to keep you from eating too little or too much of it. If you crave protein, eat more. If the thought of one more egg makes you cringe, eat less. There are certain people who benefit from getting more than 20 percent of their daily calories from protein. These include people who need to lose a considerable amount of weight and are often leptin and/or insulin resistant, those who are stressed (including people on heavy exercise regimens and who don't get enough sleep), and people who are getting older and are suffering from muscle wasting.

The exact number of protein grams that you should eat each day varies greatly depending on your gender, age, and muscle-mass-to-fat ratio. A good general rule is to experiment with between 0.325 and 0.75 gram of protein a day per pound of body weight. This roughly corresponds to 20 percent of calories and is the right amount for most people (with the exceptions noted above) to maintain lean body mass, hormone balance, and positive nitrogen levels.[2]

GRASS-FED VERSUS GRAIN-FED MEAT

With the misleading food labels in most grocery stores, it can be very confusing to know which forms of protein are the healthiest. I'm going to make it simple for you: Organic, grass-fed meat provides more nutrients and fewer toxins than grain-fed or conventional meat, with more antioxidants, omega-3s, trace minerals, and vitamins than any other food. Consuming grass-fed meat is one of the best ways to prevent disease, improve brain function, lose weight, and become Bulletproof.

In 2006, a study measured the fatty acid composition of meat from three categories—one from cattle that were fed grains for just 80 days before slaughter, one from animals fed "by-product feedstuff" that contained a mixture of grains and a cottonseed/protein mix, and one that was exclusively grass-fed.[3] The grass-fed cows had more healthy omega-3s and more conjugated linoleic acid (CLA), which is a type of naturally occurring trans fatty acid that improves brain function, causes weight loss, and reduces your risk of cancer. Just 80 days of grain feeding was enough to destroy the omega-3 and CLA content of the beef, but the longer the animal ate grains, the lower the quality of the meat. The omega-3 quantity in grain-fed meat was so low that it didn't qualify as a meaningful dietary source, while the grass-fed meat had enough omega-3s to be considered a good source of these fats.

Good science is repeatable. In 2008, another study compared a broad spectrum of nutrients in grass-fed to those in grain-fed beef.[4] The grass-fed meat had higher levels of carotenoids, which are pigments that make the fat appear yellow. Generally, the more carotenoids in a substance, the more nutrients it contains. Yellow fat (like grass-fed butter) is a sign of high nutrient density. One of the things you'll notice when cooking grass-fed meat is the yellowish color of the fat. More carotenoids equal more antioxidants, nutrients, and flavor! The grass-fed meat had slightly less total fat than grain-fed meat, but the real difference was the type of fat in each meat. Grass-fed meat was higher in saturated fat, omega-3s, CLA, and trans-vaccenic acid, which is similar to CLA. The grain-fed and grass-fed animals had about the same amounts of omega-6s, total polyunsaturated

A few friends introduced me to Bulletproof Coffee about 9 months before I left to run across the country. At first I thought the idea of adding saturated fat to your diet was insane, but it only took trying Bulletproof Coffee one time to see there was really something to it. I gradually began switching over to the Bulletproof Diet by eliminating sugar and dairy and adding grass-fed protein and fat. When I take care of my body this way, it performs and heals more efficiently. I need my body to get me all the way across America, and I'm grateful for the Bulletproof Diet for helping me get there. —**Anna Judd, athlete/activist running across America**

fat, and cholesterol. This means the grass-fed meat had a better ratio of omega-6 to omega-3 fatty acids and healthier fats overall.

Some people assume that organic meat is just as good as grass-fed meat, but it's clear from these studies that the differences in the fat content between grass-fed and grain-fed meat were related specifically to the animal's diet. Organic grain-fed meat is certainly better than conventional meat, however, which contains obesity-causing hormones and toxins formed by mold that wind up in cattle food and get added during meat processing. If an animal isn't fed nutritious food, it won't *become* nutritious food. There is no magical transformation from stale gummy bears (sometimes part of the feedlot diet) into vitamins, minerals, and healthy fats. Feeding cattle junk food turns them into junk food. Ruminant animals are meant to eat grass, not grains, stale bread, cereal, chicken feathers, or city garbage, as are sometimes added to cut the cost of animal feed (I couldn't make this up if I tried). Grass-fed meat is better for the economy, the environment, the farmers, and the animals. But most important and relevant to this book—it's far better for you.

MOM WAS RIGHT—
EAT YOUR VEGETABLES

The Bulletproof Diet is high in nutrient-rich vegetables. Read that twice, please—it does not say "fruits and vegetables." As you read in the previous chapter, fruit is full of performance-sapping fructose and should only be eaten in small amounts. Vegetables, however, are extremely healthy, and on the Bulletproof Diet you should eat as many vegetables as you can possibly stand. When it comes to vegetables, you can't eat too many. If you were to translate this into FDA servings, which vary greatly due to the vegetable's water content, it would come to 6 to 11 servings of vegetables per day. If this seems like too much food on top of the fat and protein I already mentioned, that's fine! If you feel like eating less, that's a good thing. Don't force yourself to meet these guidelines. There is a range to all of these recommendations for a reason. For example, if you eat 70 percent of your daily calories from fat, you may need slightly less protein than someone who gets only 50 percent of their calories from fat. Because vegetables are naturally low in calories, you'll eat more servings of vegetables per day than any other food group on the Bulletproof Diet, but only 20 percent of your daily calories actually come from vegetables.

Not all veggies are created equal. Because you'll be eating so many of them, the Bulletproof Diet focuses on vegetables with the highest nutrient content and lowest antinutrient load. This will provide all of your micronutrient needs that don't come from animal products, leaving very little need to consume foods that are overloaded with sugar and refined carbohydrates. And don't worry—if you don't like vegetables, remember that you get to coat them in sea salt and delicious grass-fed butter!

JUST ENOUGH STARCH AND A LITTLE FRUIT FOR FUN

STARCH

On the Bulletproof Diet, only 5 percent of your daily calories should come from fruit and starch combined, and if losing weight is your priority you should avoid them on most days as described in the 14-day program. By getting so many micronutrients from high-quality proteins, fats, and vegetables, you'll dramatically reduce (but not completely eliminate) your need to consume Bulletproof starches such as white rice and starchy vegetables like sweet potatoes, yams, carrots, and pumpkins. When you eat zero carbs for more than a few days straight, you run the risk of being so low on carbohydrates that your body doesn't even have the amount of sugar it needs for basic physiological processes. This is a matter of debate in ketogenic-dieting circles, where some people (including guests on the *Bulletproof Radio* podcast) have thrived on near-zero-carbohydrate diets for months straight. One of the first symptoms of cutting too many carbs for too long is having very dry eyes. Being this low in carbs will also ruin your quality of sleep. You don't want to get that low. Eating no carbs for extended periods can also damage your thyroid,[5] and my history of low-carb dieting is one of the reasons I had so many thyroid issues before hacking the Bulletproof Diet. To maintain your weight or after heavy exercise, one or two servings of carbohydrates a day will keep you from getting too low on carbs while getting all the benefits of low-carb dieting. To actively lose weight, fewer carbs does help.

There is a specific type of starch called resistant starch that can radically change your gut biome and cause it to produce a beneficial fatty acid called butyrate. Some of you may have seen Richard Nikoley's mind-blowing posts on resistant starch on his popular blog, *Free the Animal,* which is where I first learned about it. Resistant starch acts more like a fiber or prebiotic than a typical starch. A prebiotic is the food that your gut bacteria eat, while a probiotic is the gut bacteria themselves. The term "resistant starch" comes from the fact that these starches are resistant to digestion. This type of starch is interesting because, since your body is incapable of breaking it down, it's a starch you can eat that doesn't cause your insulin to rise and produce the resulting blood sugar problems. For some (but not all) people, resistant starch feeds the healthy bacteria in their gut. Because resistant starch does not digest in the stomach, it arrives in the colon intact. According to several studies,[6] good bacteria in the colon thrive on resistant starch and produce a short-chain fatty acid called butyrate (butyric acid) when they digest it. Butyrate is vital for a healthy gut and a healthy brain, both when you digest it and produce it. One reason that butter is so Bulletproof is that it is high in butyric acid!

I don't recommend you experiment with resistant starch during the 14-day Bulletproof Diet plan because it can have all sorts of unpredictable impacts and can take 6 weeks or more to adjust to having it in your diet. One emerging theory is that if your stomach isn't able to handle resistant starch, you may have imbalanced gut bacteria. This is likely if you've taken antibiotics in the past year or eat industrial meat. You can get a gastrointestinal pathogen panel or even have the genetic sequencing of your gut bacteria done (I've done both!) to work on that problem. This is a biohack that may well be worth your time, but it takes work beyond the scope of this book to implement properly and likely requires specific probiotics to work. That said, some people find that including resistant starch in their diets can hack the gut biome and improve their overall health. Another benefit of resistant starch is that when taken at night, it can stabilize blood sugar and provide building blocks for serotonin, helping you sleep better.

The main types of resistant starch don't exist in most typical diets. They include green banana flour, plantain flour, a special kind of resistant cornstarch, and potato starch. Some people respond better to some of these forms of resistant starch than others, so it's a good idea to try all four and see what works best for you. Because so many people's gut biomes can't handle resistant starch, it's not included in the 2-week Bulletproof Diet. Two weeks on the Bulletproof Diet will improve your gut biome anyway, and once you're in maintenance mode your gut may benefit even more from including it. The research on resistant starch is brandnew, and you can expect to see a lot more written about this in the coming months and years. But you can benefit now by becoming your own biohacker and seeing which forms of resistant starch (if any) work for you.

Don't despair if, after you finish the 14-day plan, you try eating resistant starch only to find it causes you to have endless flatulence and discomfort. This has been the case for me with most forms of resistant starch despite some advanced biohacking experimentation and consultation with experts. It turns out that there is another way to feed healthy gut bacteria and make butyric acid in the gut that is largely unknown in Western diets—consuming gelatin, collagen, and connective tissue from meat (think ribs!). I feel and perform better on these foods than I do on resistant starch, but individual genetics, your gut biome, and even the physical structure of your gut may be influencers here. Now that you know this, be a biohacker and see if resistant starch or gelatin works better for you. Whichever one you end up with, keep eating gelatin or collagen because they're vital protein sources!

Whether you consume the Bulletproof starches on the 2-week plan, resistant starch, and/or collagen, it is important to feed your gut bacteria something. While I was developing the Bulletproof Diet, I heard that some Eskimo populations survived on no carbohydrates at all, and I decided to try this to see what it would do to my health and performance. The result of that experiment was a host of new food allergies because the bacteria in my gut were literally starving, and my body did not have enough carbohydrate to efficiently maintain my gut lining. Most people are going to be better off with both resistant starch and gelatin in addition to one or two servings of starchy vegetables every day or two on the Bulletproof Diet. Sadly, a diet of only steak and butter won't work for the long term, even though it works great for several days at a time.

FRUITS

Fruits have a small amount of fiber and a few nutrients, but the amount of sugar (particularly fructose) they contain makes them a good dessert option rather than a healthy diet staple. On the Bulletproof Diet, you should eat no more than 25 grams of fructose a day, which is roughly the amount in about two apples. As you'll read later in the book, the most Bulletproof fruits are those with the least fructose, the most nutrients, and the lowest risk of antinutrients and mold toxin contamination. These include raspberries, blackberries, and strawberries.

THE MAIN SOURCES OF NUTRITIONAL KRYPTONITE

On the Bulletproof Diet, there is a set of specific Kryptonite foods that are not worth putting in your body. They provide little or no benefits while making you fat, sluggish, and weak. Later we'll talk about the individual foods you should strive to avoid, but first let's discuss the main types of food that I consider Kryptonite. While you're enjoying delicious fats and high-quality proteins along with plenty of veggies and low-to-moderate amounts of carbs, here are the food groups you won't miss.

PERFORMANCE-SAPPING SUGAR

You've already read about how fructose makes you fat, raises your tri-glycerides, ages your tissues, and saps your willpower. Regular table sugar is half fructose and half glucose. That means it's less harmful than pure fructose or high-fructose corn syrup, which has undergone processing to change some of its glucose to fructose to make it sweeter. Fructose raises tri-glycerides more than regular sugar does and as a result causes more meta-bolic damage, but the problem with regular sugar is that, unlike fructose, it triggers the same reward centers in many people's brains that cocaine does. But sugar is legal, and it's everywhere. There's even evidence that consuming a lot of sugar can decrease the number of dopamine receptors in your brain,[7] making it harder for you to feel the energy and pleasure from your body's production of dopamine. This is called dopamine resistance. The same exact thing happens to drug addicts! To top it off, sugar provides zero satiation, so you're left hungry immediately after consuming large amounts of it.

Eating sugar makes you tired, disrupts brain and hormone function, and promotes obesity. Most people are familiar with the term "sugar crash," but many don't know where this term comes from. After you eat sugar, it's not only your focus and energy that crash, but also your actual blood sugar levels, too. Insulin is a hormone secreted by the pancreas that regulates blood sugar. When you eat sugar, blood sugars naturally rise, causing the pancreas to secrete insulin. But the pancreas isn't great at estimating how much insulin to release and usually overdoes it, secreting large amounts of insulin that cause your blood sugar to drop dramatically. *This* is the famous crash that causes brain fog, sluggishness, and food cravings. When the crash comes, the Labrador in your head feels like your body is starving, and it reduces energy to your human brain right when you need it to apply more willpower to make the Labrador behave. The result? You find yourself eating the cookie you swore you weren't going to eat.

When insulin levels are boosted from eating sugar and excess carbohydrates, your body gets the signal to store fat instead of burning it. This is because insulin regulates blood sugar levels by moving excess glucose into fat cells, where they are stored with water as saturated fat. When insulin levels are kept low on the Bulletproof Diet, your body has no fuel to burn except fat, so it does so consistently and efficiently. The consumption of excess sugar and carbohydrates is a major factor in the obesity epidemic, and eliminating sugar is one of the very best things you can do for your health, weight, and overall performance.

POISONOUS PROCESSED FOODS

As a young adult, I really enjoyed eating gyros, Greek sandwiches containing roasted meat, at a restaurant near my office. After I learned that I felt better when I avoided gluten, I asked them to slice the meat directly onto a big salad and serve it without any bread. I thought this made for a nice, healthy lunch, but I started to experience severe brain fog 2 hours after lunch, and after experimenting with different meals I correlated that specific lunch with the unwanted foggy feeling. I went to the restaurant and asked the cook what was in the meat, and I found out that the nice rotisserie meat I was eating also contained soy protein, monosodium glutamate (MSG), and other strange ingredients that weren't actually meat. The food I was eating had been processed and manipulated by the restaurant in order to make the more expensive meat stretch further, and it was those additives that were causing me to lag in the afternoon. When my Labrador brain demanded an energy boost 2 hours after lunch, I started a terrible habit of eating sugar and drinking more coffee in the late afternoon to

> I tried to lose weight by jogging three times a week, but after 6 months I'd barely dropped 10 pounds. Within weeks of hearing about the Bulletproof Diet, I went sugar-, dairy-, and gluten-free and started drinking Bulletproof Coffee at least four times a week. I lost almost 50 pounds, and my doctor told me to keep doing whatever I was doing. I plan to hike the Pacific Crest Trail and to stay Bulletproof through the hike. I've been doing practice hikes this summer. I substitute ghee for the butter and add a little almond cacao butter with the Brain Octane, and it really hits the spot before a day's hike. **—Jeffrey**

keep me going. But when I avoided eating the chemical meat for lunch, I didn't need the extra boost later.

The same thing happens with energy bars and other foods that have been processed to include inexpensive proteins, chemically damaged fats, and synthetic flavorings. MSG is one of the most common artificial flavorings added to processed foods. MSG is a chemical that is meant to make food taste better. It was developed in Japan during World War II to help sell lower-quality or even spoiled foods. By making things that really weren't food taste good, MSG helped food producers sell empty calories to consumers. And it does taste good, but MSG also messes with the way your neurotransmitters cause the nerves in your brain to fire. MSG is an excitatory neurotransmitter that sends signals from one cell to another. Consuming it can cause the cells it activates to become overexcited. This leads to cell damage and often cell death. As your cells become damaged and/or die, your neurons signal for more energy. You may experience this as a headache, a sudden mood swing, or a craving for sweets, the fastest source of energy. This is obviously a substance to avoid for optimum performance! The most common sources of MSG are processed chips, commercial salad dressings, broths, commercial soups, and sauces like barbecue sauce and ketchup. Most spice mixes also contain MSG.

Artificial sweeteners are another common additive in processed foods, especially "sugar free" snack foods. Aspartame is one synthetic sweetener that is responsible for a large number of adverse reactions. I used to consume aspartame before I became aware of how harmful it is. I enjoyed its sweet taste and thought I was doing myself a favor by drinking diet soda (which contains aspartame) instead of regular soda. But I was wrong. Both MSG and aspartame caused my blood sugar levels to fluctuate so badly that it took years for me to sort them out. Because they don't contain any real sugar or calories, it was hard to pin down aspartame and MSG as the causes of those blood sugar swings. Now that I'm aware, it's amazing to realize what a stick of sugar-free gum with aspartame does to my performance!

Aspartame, which is now marketed as AminoSweet as well as Nutra-Sweet, is made of two amino acids, which are protein's building blocks. These amino acids wouldn't be harmful if one of them, phenylalanine, wasn't chemically altered. (Pardon the slight detour into biochemistry here.) The addition of a methyl ester bond to phenylalanine makes it taste sweet, but the side effect is that it makes it easy for phenylalanine to form free methanol (wood alcohol). There is methanol in vegetables and fruits, but when found there it's bound to pectin and doesn't harm you. When methanol is free, it gets converted into formaldehyde in the liver.[8] This is just as poisonous to your body as it sounds. Aspartame can cause long-term damage and doesn't belong in your diet if you are interested in feeling amazing, living a long time, or performing anywhere near your best.

There are several other sweet food additives that provide no benefit and contain significant risks, including acesulfame K (ace-K), saccharin, sucralose (Splenda), and tagatose. By eating mostly high-quality fats, protein, and vegetables on the Bulletproof Diet, it will be easy for you to avoid these ingredients without having to waste time reading ingredient lists on packages of processed Kryptonite foods. Don't worry—there are safe sweeteners you can use on the Bulletproof Diet and even recipes later in the book for delicious, sweet, and satisfying Bulletproof desserts.

GMO INGREDIENTS

People often don't think of GMO ingredients as processed foods, but if you define "processed" as chemically altered, then GMOs are indeed as processed as any other Frankenfood. The term "genetically modified" means that either a crop or an animal's genes have been altered for some specific purpose. Unfortunately, GMO foods are becoming ubiquitous, especially among canola, corn, cottonseed, sugar cane, potatoes, and soy crops. While some people disagree, I consider the products made with these ingredients, such as vegetable oils and high-fructose corn syrup, to be Kryptonite.

Consuming GMOs is so unproven and risky that a few countries have outlawed the practice of GMO farming, while most require GMO foods to be clearly labeled. But in the United States, GMO farming is not only allowed, there is also no law requiring food labels to state whether or not they contain GMO ingredients. In the United States, if a food is labeled "organic" it cannot contain any GMO ingredients, so the best way to avoid GMO ingredients completely is to purchase only certified organic food.

As GMOs have become popular over the past 3 decades, there has also been a 400 percent increase in allergies, a 300 percent increase in asthma, a 400 percent increase in attention deficit/hyperactivity disorder, and a 1,500 percent increase in autism spectrum disorder.[9] The science is still out as to whether or not there's a definite connection between GMOs and these health issues, but until these foods are proven to be safe I recommend avoiding them. This may be controversial in the United States, but in the rest of the world people are aware of the risks of consuming GMOs. There, they are widely believed to cause reproductive issues, immune dysfunction, and a host of other issues. Regardless of the other possible health risks, it is certain that GMOs contain far fewer nutrients than their non-GMO equivalents. There is simply no reason to eat GMO foods if you want to be a high-performing individual.

VEGETABLE OILS
THAT DON'T COME FROM VEGETABLES

The Bulletproof Diet is all about fat, but the type of fat you consume is key. As you read earlier, the most stable fats are saturated, while the most unstable, easily oxidized, and therefore inflammatory fats are polyunsaturated fats. Eating excess polyunsaturated fats will not improve your health, longevity, or performance and is likely to contribute to cancer and metabolic problems. The most common polyunsaturated oils that you should avoid include canola, corn, cottonseed, peanut, safflower, soybean, sunflower, and all other vegetable oils. Besides being so unstable, the main problems with these oils are that most are genetically modified and many contain toxic solvents used in their production. It's not easy to squeeze oil out of something like corn, so in order to maximize production, solvents are needed. As a result, these oils cause inflammation rather than reducing it like healthier Bulletproof fats like grass-fed animal fat, coconut oil, Brain Octane Oil, butter, or olive oil do.

These Kryptonite oils also provide unhealthy amounts of omega-6 polyunsaturated fats. Your body does need omega-6s, but we eat so many of them in a standard Western diet that it's almost impossible to consume too few. Ideally, you should consume no more than four times as many omega-6s as omega-3s, but most people today eat 20 to 50 times as many omega-6s. This is important because an imbalance in tissue fatty acid content is one of the most potent sources of inflammation, as omega-6 is proinflammatory and normal levels of omega-3 are anti-inflammatory.

If you eat the oils that most restaurants and processed food companies use, you're getting huge amounts of an inflammatory omega-6 fatty acid called linoleic acid, way more than humans have ever consumed in history. It is not benign. Linoleic acid and other omega-6 oils are incorporated into your cell membranes and are even stored as body fat. Since these oils are unstable, they oxidize in your body (not to mention when you cook them). Oxidized omega-6 fats do damage to your DNA, inflame your heart tissues, and raise your risk of several types of cancer including breast cancer. But perhaps worst of all, your brain pays the price—oxidized omega-6 fats don't support optimal brain metabolism.[10] Anything that increases general inflammation in the body isn't going to help your brain perform better, and excess omega-6 fats are no exception.

When these oils are used in packaged foods, they are usually stabilized in order to sit on the shelf by a process called hydrogenation. This process, which turns already unhealthy fats into more harmful synthetic trans fats, has been linked to many health problems and is a major cause of obesity. The government has made efforts to reduce, but not eliminate, hydrogenated oils. When you ingest man-made trans fats, your body tries to use them to build cells, but cell walls made of these trans fats cannot function properly. There is one naturally occurring trans fat that is chemically completely different from artificial trans fats. It is called conjugated linoleic acid (CLA, mentioned earlier in the chapter) and is found in grass-fed butter. While artificial trans fats damage your health and performance, CLA has a host of health benefits. It is absolutely not the same as margarine.

GUT-DESTROYING GRAINS

Wheat is a particularly important grain to avoid because of the many negative side effects of gluten, a protein found in wheat and other grains. As I mentioned before, the first time I lost a substantial amount of weight (about 50 pounds) was after going on a standard low-carb diet. In addition to losing weight, I found that my personality changed dramatically. I'm not proud of this, but I'll own up to the fact that as an obese young man, I had overdeveloped muscles in my middle finger because of road rage. After I went on the low-carb diet and ditched the gluten, my family noticed that I was far less angry than usual, and my Labrador brain's desire to flip off other drivers magically went away. It felt like I was waking up from a fog.

It was clear to me that something in my diet had caused these drastic personality changes, and as I experimented with adding different types of carbs back in, I quickly saw that it was gluten. As the Bulletproof Diet began to take shape, I started doing a "cheat day" once a week. On that day, I'd often eat gluten. Tracking my energy, mood, and food cravings, I noticed that when I ate gluten I was fine the day after, but 2 or 3 days later

I became cranky and foggy. Although this is unusual, some people respond to a food exposure up to 10 days later. This may be because it takes a while for inflammation to travel through the body and reach the brain. For me, eating gluten on Saturday night meant brain fog Monday morning.

Gluten-containing grains are addictive and break down in the gut into opioid compounds called gluteomorphins that trigger the same receptors in your brain as opiate drugs like heroin. If allow your Labrador brain to get "addicted" to the opiates formed by grain digestion, your human brain is going to experience that as insatiable hunger and cravings that last for days after you last ate grains. Every single piece of bread will have a siren call that sucks your willpower until you give in and eat it.

I struggled with this problem for years. I'd give up gluten and grains only to have "just one piece" on a cheat day. Then the next day my Labrador brain would trick me into rationalizing the case for eating "just one more." Soon I was on the slippery slope of gluten-induced weight gain and brain fog. Opiate addicts don't have "just one," and you shouldn't eat any gluten-containing grains, either. The trick is to give them up completely. This will dramatically increase your ability to live up to your full potential and you'll undoubtedly feel an immediate difference in your body and your brain.

There is plenty of research to show that eating gluten has negative health consequences. It causes inflammation and gastrointestinal distress

In 2012, I was diagnosed with multiple sclerosis. I was told that it is a degenerative disease and the quality of my life will get worse and worse. I did my own research, and all of my remaining symptoms were gone within 3 days of starting the Bulletproof Diet. They have not come back. I can't imagine how my life would be now if I hadn't made the changes that I did. I can honestly say I've never been healthier in my life. I am currently enrolled at the Institute of Integrative Nutrition, and I hope to help and inspire as many people as I can. —**Josh** and contributes to autoimmune diseases and a host of other issues. Gluten causes overrelease of zonulin, a protein that controls the spaces between your gut cells. When the gap between your intestinal cells opens after eating gluten, bacteria, undigested food, and toxins flood into your bloodstream. This causes inflammation throughout your entire body, including in your brain. Gluten also reduces blood flow to the brain and can interfere with thyroid function.[11] In one study, feeding wheat to healthy volunteers depleted their vitamin D stores.[12] Perhaps worst of all, the effects of gluten exposure can last for up to 6 months in your immune system. While some people have a more extreme reaction than others, this goes for everyone, not just those who are sensitive to gluten.

No doubt about it, grains are great at keeping people alive when there is no other food available, such as in times of food scarcity. Eating grains is much better than starving during a famine. But when societies begin growing grain, especially wheat, they experience skeletal deformities, particularly in the jaw and spine, and the average height goes down over multiple generations.[13] There are plenty of other reasons to avoid most grains. As I explained earlier, antinutrients (particularly mold toxins, lectins, and phytates) are common in most grains, beans, and seeds. Corn is a double whammy, as it frequently contains mold toxins (from a *Fusarium* species that infects corn as it grows) and is often genetically modified. Another indirect problem with corn is that these days most farmed animals eat a great deal of corn in addition to other garbage and foods lacking nutrients, as it is cheap and easy for farmers to produce. But consuming animals that eat corn is sometimes even more harmful than eating the corn itself, as many animals concentrate the corn toxins in their fat. Corn and its derivative products are Kryptonite and are found in almost all processed foods. It will keep you from starving, but it won't help you thrive.

DUBIOUS DAIRY

The final category of foods to avoid on the Bulletproof Diet is conventional dairy. This includes milk and most things made from milk—

cheese, yogurt, cream, buttermilk, and ice cream—but not butter or its cleaner cousin, ghee (clarified butter). Butter is significantly healthier than the milk it is made from because the harmful milk proteins (including casein and BCM-7) are largely absent from butter. What little milk protein remains in cultured butter has been enzymatically modified during the butter fermentation process and isn't a problem for most people. Most people can eat plenty of grass-fed butter and feel Bulletproof, but if you have a slight allergy to casein and lactose, you can switch to ghee, which doesn't contain either. I'm actually allergic to dairy protein, but I can happily eat butter—and plenty of it—without a problem. Butter is also low in mold toxins. Less than 2 percent of even conventional butter is contaminated with mycotoxins.[14] It's the dairy protein, casein, that concentrates mycotoxins.

The secret ingredient in butter that makes it so good for you is butyrate, the same compound your gut bacteria produce when you eat resistant starch. Butyrate is a short-chain saturated fatty acid that has profound effects in obese mice fed a high-fat diet—it lowered blood cholesterol by 25 percent and cut triglycerides, then increased insulin sensitivity by a whopping 300 percent. It also prevented obesity, increased body temperature, and had a huge impact on improving mitochondrial function. Yes, a fat found in butter did that in mice . . . and seemed to have done the same types of things in me. In humans, butyrate has been proven to reduce inflammation[15] even in the brain, and it keeps toxins from penetrating the gut lining, too.

A 2014 study found that eating butyrate was associated with an increased amount of healthy bacteria in the gut.[16] We used to believe that butyrate created by fermentation in the lower gut was the same as butyrate from your diet, but this study showed that eating the short-chain fatty acids found in butter may affect the health of your lower GI tract in a slightly different way. This means it's not enough to either produce butyrate or eat it—to get the best results, you have to do both.

Not all butter is created equal, however. Your butter must come from grass-fed cows in order to provide you with all of its potential health benefits, including 500 IU of vitamin A, more carotenes than carrots, and high amounts of vitamins K_2, D, and E in just 1 tablespoon of grass-fed butter. If you're not yet convinced that butter is actually a health food, take a moment to consider this one fact: In 1910, butter consumption was 18 pounds per capita and heart disease rates were below 10 percent. In 2000, butter consumption was less than 4 pounds per capita and heart disease killed 40 to 45 percent of people.

Conventional dairy products have surprisingly little in common with butter or ghee. One of the main problems with dairy is the harmful process of pasteurization, which heats milk to 150°F for about 30 minutes before it is stored at temperatures below 55°F. This process does reduce the small risk of milk contamination, but it also kills off the beneficial probiotics in the milk, denatures milk proteins, and basically transforms milk from a source of nutrition into a source of many health problems.

In addition to reducing the vitamin content in milk, pasteurization turns milk's lactose sugars into beta-lactose sugars that the body absorbs faster, causing blood sugar spikes. Pasteurization also transforms the calcium in milk so that the human body cannot absorb it[17] and alters milk's primary protein, casein, so that it is difficult to properly digest. Amazingly, the medical community has known about the harmful effects of pasteurization since the 1930s when children who drank raw (unpasteurized) milk were found to have less tooth decay than children who drank pasteurized milk.[18]

But pasteurization isn't the only harmful way milk is processed. In raw milk, the cream separates from the rest of the milk and naturally rises to the top. Homogenization is a process that prevents the cream from separating, making milk more stable for store shelves. But this practice also has harmful effects. All milk naturally contains a potentially harmful enzyme called xanthine oxidase (XO), but when you drink non-homogenized milk, your body is able to efficiently break down the XO and keep it out of the bloodstream. When milk is homogenized, globules of fat surround the XO, making it impossible for your body to break it down, with unknown effects.

Cheese is even more problematic than milk because the very process that turns milk into cheese also promotes the buildup of toxins. All cheeses are made using a combination of yeast, other fungi, and/or bacteria that form toxins in the cheese that kill off other organisms. But these toxins are also harmful to humans in varying degrees. Each and every batch of cheese may contain a unique mix of fungi from its environment, so it's nearly impossible to know exactly which toxins the cheese you're eating contains. The safest bet is to avoid cheeses altogether, as mold toxins are found in more than 40 percent of conventionally produced cheeses.[19] The casein in cheese also concentrates the mold toxins consumed in the animal's diet. The process of pasteurizing cheese causes all the same problems as pasteurizing milk, particularly high amounts of denatured (less digestible, damaged) casein.

Other than butter and ghee, which are Bulletproof, the only form of dairy I recommend is a Suspect food that may or may not work for you—full-fat organic raw milk, kefir, or yogurt from grass-fed cows. If you test yourself and can tolerate these, they can be a great addition to your diet. Low-temperature-processed, grass-fed whey protein concentrate also works well for some people, but use no more than 2 to 4 tablespoons per day, as whey is high in amino acids that can cause inflammation in excess.

The good news is that it is not necessary to consume dairy protein in any form on the Bulletproof Diet because you'll get the same health benefits from other delicious Bulletproof foods without any of the risks.

FUEL YOUR BRAIN

Studies show that when you work a region of the brain harder, the microcapillaries deliver more blood to that part of the brain,[20] and when it gets there, the neurons actually use the energy delivered in the blood.[21] The implication, which is still a matter of debate in academia, is that cutting calories can negatively impact your brain function as well as your body, while feeding your body with more calories actually provides you with more brainpower. This is a scientific explanation of something that feels pretty obvious when you think about it. I know I don't think particularly well when I'm hungry!

A calorie deficit is definitely a stressor on your body, and nonproductive stress lowers brain function. You will not function in an optimal state for very long if you aren't eating enough calories, and consuming as many calories as your body demands is a critical part of the Bulletproof Diet. As long as they come from the right sources and you're listening to your hunger, the more calories you eat, the more calories your metabolism—and brain—will use. Surprisingly, we have seen in fruit flies that severe caloric restriction, meaning consuming one-third fewer calories than the body burns, helps increase longevity. Some of my antiaging colleagues have tried this with mixed results. From looking at the research, it appears there is increasingly less evidence that this works in humans. You can get

> I wondered why I used to get stomachaches, and now I know—yogurt! The Bulletproof program made me aware. **—Dawn**

most of the genetic benefits of those regimens with a class of supplements called calorie restriction mimetics, anyway.

The Bulletproof Diet does not dictate exactly how many calories you should eat in a day, because when you stop feeding it Kryptonite foods, your body will naturally regulate how much you want to eat. Nowadays, I normally eat about 2,500 to 3,000 calories a day, and I'm a muscular 6-foot-4-inch male. If you follow the overall meal plan and eat Bulletproof foods, you won't need to worry so much about the exact number of calories you consume. If you're accustomed to following a typical American diet or have a habit of counting calories in order to lose weight, the thought of giving up this practice might be scary. These diets may have gotten you so out of tune with your body that you don't even recognize when you are hungry or when you're full, and so you rely on calorie counting and prepackaged meals to tell you how much and when to eat.

The good news is that you're finally going to be free of all that on the Bulletproof Diet. When you start eating the right amounts of good fats with adequate protein and none of the garbage that breaks your body's natural appetite-regulation equipment, your energy and hunger systems will come back online. You'll know when you're hungry and you'll know when you're satisfied. There will be no more sugar crashes and you won't have to suppress your appetite anymore.

Diets have led so many of us to not trust ourselves. You may be worried that you'll overeat and gain weight on the Bulletproof Diet, but one of the best things about this diet is that it was designed to avoid overeating. The high amounts of fat you'll be consuming are so satiating that you won't want to overeat. In fact, it's virtually impossible to overeat on high-quality fats *because* they are so satiating. If you do find yourself gaining weight on the Bulletproof Diet (which is highly unlikely, but not impossible), it's probably because you're eating too many carbs or you have hormone problems that need proper diagnosis. When you cut back on carbs and refocus on good fats, protein, and vegetables, the weight will come off effortlessly and life itself will get easier.

CHAPTER 4

EAT FAT FOR BREAKFAST AND CARBS FOR DESSERT

An interesting thing I learned through my antiaging research is that there's a rhythm to the body's sodium and potassium requirements. Your body needs more sodium than potassium in the morning so your blood pressure can go up, but eating fruit (which has a lot of potassium) for breakfast causes your blood pressure to go down. Low blood pressure in the morning makes it harder to feel energized and ready to face the day. This was the first time I realized that eating (or avoiding) specific foods at certain times of day could cause a desired reaction in the body.

Though I wasn't eating fruit for breakfast when I followed the extremely low-carb Eskimo diet for 3 months, I noticed that I woke up every morning feeling exhausted. My sleep-tracking apps (which I'll talk about more later) showed that I was waking up nine times a night. For me, optimizing sleep was particularly important, and my research told me that sustained low-carb diets negatively impact sleep because the brain needs some glucose to operate efficiently while asleep. In 2011, I met the late Seth Roberts at a Quantified Self conference, where people who are interested in self-tracking or biohacking gather to share ideas. Seth Roberts was a Quantified Self pioneer who did some great research on butter, and made a convincing case for eating at least a few carbohydrates in the evening for sleep quality.

Why do so many of us eat granola and fruit in the morning? Because a company selling those products told us to. But the science shows us that the best time to eat those foods isn't when you may think. The idea that you can eat the same food at a different time of day to get a different reaction from your body flies in the face of the idea that counting calories is all you need to do to lose weight. But is it really so odd when you think about it? Some cultures have known about this for centuries. During Ramadan, the month designated by the Islamic calendar as the 9th in the year, Muslims fast during the day and then eat as much as they want at night, while Ayurvedic medicine has recognized the benefits of partial-day fasting for thousands of years. By researching these traditions and the body's circadian rhythms and then experimenting on myself, I came up with a few simple timing hacks that will make a dramatic difference in the way you look, feel, sleep, and perform. It all starts with the most important meal (or in my case, beverage) of the day—breakfast.

BULLETPROOF COFFEE

I first learned about the power of blended butter from a tiny Tibetan woman at 18,300 feet of elevation in a remote part of Tibet near Mt. Kailash. In 2004, I staggered into her guesthouse chilled from the thin, −10°F air and she rejuvenated me with a creamy cup of traditional yak butter tea. I couldn't get enough of it. The biohacker in me asked, "Why does drinking this stuff make me feel so good even though there's no air? And why would a nomadic person who lives in a tent and must pack light bother to carry a heavy blender or a hand churn?" These questions were a part of the genesis of the Bulletproof Coffee recipe.

When I returned home I brewed some tea, tossed it in the blender with some butter, and experienced nothing but a greasy cup of tea. Clearly, something different was happening back in Tibet. I picked up some high-end tea from a local Chinese merchant, but it still didn't have the magical effect I remembered. So I went to my local Whole Foods and another gourmet store, where I bought every single brand of gourmet butter from around the world to see if the butter was the variable that mattered. It was. After trying each of them, I learned that the trick was to use unsalted butter from grass-fed cows. If you're lucky, you can get it from a local farmer, but for the rest of us, Kerrygold Pure Irish Butter (in the United States and European Union) and the New Zealand–produced Anchor Butter (in much of Asia and Australia) fits the bill.

From my antiaging research I knew about the tremendous health benefits of coconut oil, so I began experimenting with adding coconut milk and coconut oil to the tea, but it overwhelmed the tea. I switched from tea to coffee, my other great love (besides butter, of course). The coffee stood up to the coconut oil better than tea, and the final crowning achievement was to add 1 or 2 teaspoons of Brain Octane Oil (a coconut extract) to the coffee along with 1 or 2 teaspoons of unsalted, grass-fed butter or ghee. Together, these ingredients created the creamiest, most delicious, best performance-boosting cup of coffee I'd ever experienced. This is Bulletproof Coffee. For more than 7 years, I have started each and every day with a cup of Bulletproof Coffee, using the extra energy and brainpower it provides to hack my body while blowing the doors off my career and thriving in every area of my life. It turned my brain back on and freed me from food cravings, and it's done the same thing for tens of thousands of others.

The full Bulletproof Coffee recipe was able to keep me thin even when I was trying to gain fat on a diet of more than 4,000 calories a day with no exercise. I was determined to fully understand why. The first beneficial component of coffee is caffeine. Caffeine itself from any source is more than an energy booster. It may help ease cognitive decline and lower the risk of developing Alzheimer's disease by blocking inflammation in the brain.[1] According to Gregory Freund, MD, from the University of

Illinois, "We have discovered a novel signal that activates the brain-based inflammation associated with neurodegenerative diseases, and caffeine appears to block its activity."[2] Caffeine also increases insulin sensitivity in healthy humans,[3,4] which is extremely important to sustained weight loss.

Drinking any coffee has short- and long-term effects on your brain. The short-term effect of coffee on mood may be due to altered serotonin and dopamine activity, whereas the mechanisms behind its potential long-term effects on mood may relate to its antioxidant and anti-inflammatory proper-ties.[5,6,7] But as you read earlier, the type of coffee you drink is also incredibly important. I can feel a negative change in how my brain works when I have moldy coffee, which is what led me to work on solving the problem with pre-dictable results. I started lab testing coffee to identify the agricultural prac-tices that led to perfectly clean beans that consistently gave me the highest performance. It took 10 years to identify every step of performance-robbing toxin formation in coffee in the way it's grown, harvested, and shipped, and to create a reliable, perfect source of beans that always make you feel great when "normal" coffee gives you headaches, jitters, and crankiness.

After lab testing my own beans for toxins, I asked volunteers to try them and see if there was a noticeable difference. The response was really positive, but I knew it was possible that it was all a placebo effect—meaning that they may have felt a difference simply because they expected to feel a difference. To shed some light on this, I designed a study to determine what

> About 2 months ago, I was hit with a bout of adrenal fatigue. In the pro-cess of doing some online searches, I came across the Bulletproof Web site. This has been an incredible discovery. Coffee is supposed to be avoided if you have adrenal fatigue, but I ordered a Bulletproof kit with coffee beans and Brain Octane. I start my day this way along with a glass of water with Himalayan salt and a 15-minute yoga posture. This regimen has propelled me ahead in my recovery. The first question I ask myself now before I eat or drink anything is, Is it Bulletproof? Your Web site is a treasure trove of valuable information that comes across to me as a labor of love. —Don

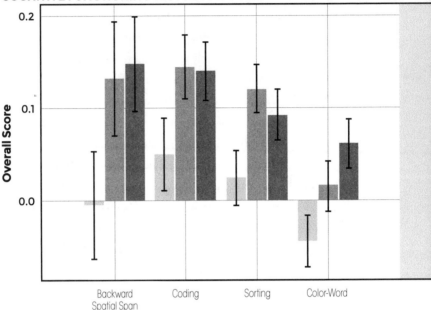

impact, if any, my mold-tested beans would have compared to coffee from local coffee shops. It was these results that confirmed what I'd discovered myself and verified with a few guinea pig friends. To do this test, I started by registering with an institutional review board, which issues approvals for tests conducted on humans to verify that they're safe. I worked with a Stanford researcher to put together a statistically valid, uncomfortably rigorous set of tests. We asked 54 people, recruited from the Bulletproof Executive Facebook page, to conduct two batteries of cognitive function tests per day for 4 weeks while using different combinations of butter and coffee:

> Lab-tested Upgraded Coffee (black)
> Coffee made with beans from a local shop (black)
> Lab-tested Upgraded Coffee with butter
> Coffee made with beans from a local shop with butter

We did not test Brain Octane Oil, short-chain MCTs, or coconut oil because the test was already too long and dropout (people not completing the test) was a problem. Nonetheless, the results were conclusive. With or

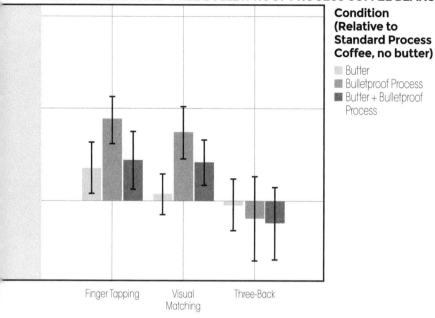

Condition (Relative to Standard Process Coffee, no butter)

▨ Butter
■ Bulletproof Process
■ Butter + Bulletproof Process

Finger Tapping   Visual Matching   Three-Back

without butter, the coffee from a local coffee shop produced statistically significant lower scores on tests of cognitive function compared to lab-tested Upgraded Coffee beans.

We measured seven different executive functions using standardized psychology tests (called backward spatial span, coding, sorting, color-word, finger tapping, visual matching, and three-back.) On six of seven measures, the lab-tested Upgraded Coffee beans increased executive function compared to commonly available coffee beans sourced from multiple regions in the United States. Surprisingly, butter had a weaker effect and even a negative effect in one test in which coffee did not have a strong effect, either. Butter works because it turns off hunger and frees up willpower, although it doesn't directly stimulate the brain the way coffee does. But thankfully, it doesn't appear to slow you down, either!

Clearly, using the right ingredients is important, but how you make your Bulletproof Coffee also has an impact on your health and performance. Certain oils in coffee—kahweol and cafestol—are unique and potent neurological anti-inflammatory agents that protect against oxidative

OVERALL COGNITIVE FUNCTIONING USING COMMODITY COFFEE BEANS VERSUS MOLD-FREE BULLETPROOF PROCESS COFFEE BEANS

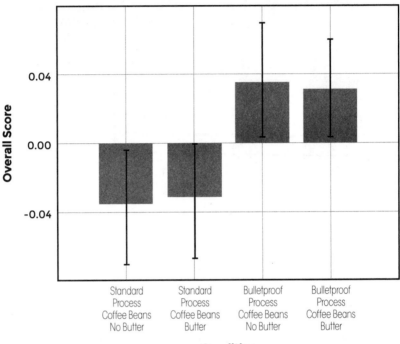

stress and DNA damage.[8] By brewing coffee with a metal filter like a French press, gold filter, or espresso machine, you save these precious coffee oils so they can do their job in your body.[9] It's also important to blend the butter and Brain Octane Oil into your coffee rather than stirring it because blending the butter breaks it up into something called micelles, which allow your body to use fat for energy. Your bile produces micelles, too, but the more of them you have, the more fat your body can use. This means blending butter into your coffee assists your body in using fat as a source of energy. If you peel back the wrapper on a stick of butter and eat it like a Snickers bar alongside a cup of coffee, the results are not the same. I should know—I've tried it!

Once I knew why properly prepared coffee made with my lab-tested low-toxin beans was so beneficial, it was time to take a closer look at the remaining elements of Bulletproof Coffee to find out how they were able to produce such energy-boosting, fat-burning results.

Imagine you were a computer hacker and you broke into a new computer only to find that another hacker got there first and was already in control of it. You'd want to put your own control systems in place and take action to prevent the other hacker from messing with the system. It turns out that your gut bacteria are the other hacker, and they've put systems in place to give you food cravings and cause you to store more excess fat than your body would naturally.

Your body has a finely tuned system for controlling fat-burning and storage.[10] Your liver creates a protein called fasting-induced adipose factor (FIAF). One thing FIAF does is block an enzyme called LPL (lipoprotein lipase), which tells your body to store fat. This means that when FIAF is high, your body burns additional fat, and your liver creates the right amount of FIAF according to your body's needs. The problem is that the bacteria in your gut also make FIAF, but they manipulate it for their own purposes. Gut bacteria are thought to actually suppress FIAF when you're eating a high-fat, high-sugar diet, and thus cause your body to store this fat rather than burning it. This is not to say that all gut bacteria are bad—they can be beneficial as long as you have the right ones in the right place. But too many or the wrong types can and will lead to obesity.

Luckily, there are ways to "out-hack" the other hackers. When gut bacteria are "starved" of starch or sugar, they get hungry. Hungry bacteria make FIAF and you burn fat. When gut bacteria are fed sugar or starch, they stop producing FIAF and you start storing fat.[11] Medium-chain triglycerides, and particularly the shortest of the medium-chain fats, put pressure on the population of gut bacteria, and when you use it during a fast you're actively interfering with gut bacteria's attempts to make you store extra fat. The polyphenols in coffee also act as a probiotic for Bacteroidetes, the phylum of bacteria found more frequently in thin people (see Chapter 1). You can't increase the population of that bacteria with supplements; you have to feed it.

By taking coffee with fat, you temporarily suppress all gut bacteria and then provide food for the "thin people" bacteria so they can proliferate. This is something I can actually see in my own gut lab panels and in Bulletproof Dieters' uBiome results when they share them with me. They have above-average amounts of Bacteroidetes, the bacteria associated with being lean, and fewer of the Firmicutes phylum, associated with being obese. You should have some of both for optimal health, but changing the ratio really impacts your energy level and ability to regulate your own weight.

There's a study in rats showing that coffee in combination with a diet high in fat (even unhealthy fats) was associated with decreased body weight, adiposity, liver triglycerides, and energy intake.[12] The coffee caused more favorable body composition and helped to optimize the critical ratio of Firmicutes to Bacteroidetes. Coffee also improved circulating short-chain fatty acids, which is also good for the gut. In that study, the rats became insulin resistant, something that also happens to humans during extended very-low-carb diets. (We hack that problem by eating a meaningful amount of carbs at least once a week on the Bulletproof Diet.)

Replacing the milk in your coffee with butter is beneficial in several ways. One of the antioxidant polyphenols in coffee that helps your performance is called chlorogenic acid. When you put the milk protein casein into your coffee by adding milk, half-and-half, cream, or most fake creamers, the polyphenols become 3.4 times less bioavailable.[13] Cultured butter has very little casein, and ghee has none. This means that by switching from milk or cream to butter, you get 3.4 times more antioxidants from your coffee! As you know, butter also contains butyric acid, which can help heal the gut and directly lowers inflammation in the brain.[14]

The Brain Octane Oil in Bulletproof Coffee adds its own unique benefits to the mix. Just be sure to start slowly with Brain Octane Oil, as too much too soon can cause what Bulletproof followers commonly refer to as "disaster pants." Much better than disaster pants, ketosis is a beneficial state where your body burns fat for energy instead of sugar. Normally, your body burns carbohydrates for fuel. When it runs out of carbohydrates, it starts converting fat to glycerol for energy. The liver produces ketones as a by-product of this fat metabolism. Ketosis is a state your body enters when you have a lot of ketones in your blood and you are burning additional fat. It's possible to enter ketosis by eating a diet that's very low in carbohydrates with moderate protein and high healthy fats, but it's hard to get there and stay there. Bulletproof Coffee hacks ketosis by using the shortest medium-chain triglyceride oil (C8 MCT), which makes it easier for your body to create ketones. In one study, simply adding 2 tablespoons of this oil to the diets of healthy young men resulted in 9 percent of their brain metabolism being powered by ketones, even when the men were eating carbohydrates! Normally, you have zero brain metabolism powered by ketones after you've eaten carbohydrates. In other words, using the right C8 extract of coconut oil instead of just plain coconut oil provides a much easier path to burning more fat and feeling more energy.[15]

Most people achieve ketosis by avoiding carbs, but this is not necessary when you have Bulletproof Coffee in the morning. I've tested this by eating a whole sushi dinner with 2 cups of rice and testing my blood ketones in the morning using a blood ketone meter that's similar to a blood glucose meter. The blood test showed a blood ketone level of 0.1, when 0.6 or above means you're officially in ketosis. I drank a cup of Bulletproof Coffee with added Brain Octane Oil, and my blood ketones hit 0.7 within 30 minutes. Bulletproof Coffee on an empty stomach is a fast path to mild ketosis and brings the benefits of mental focus and reduced food cravings. With plain coconut oil and a low-carb diet, you'd need to very carefully restrict carbs for at least 3 days to reach the same level of ketosis.

A lot of people want to try making Bulletproof Coffee using beans they can find in local shops. This is possible, and though the results are not as consistent, I've come up with some ground rules for finding the highest-quality low-toxin beans. The first step is to go to the fanciest coffee shop in your neighborhood, hopefully one with its own roaster. If you don't know which one this is, use your Web browser to search for a coffee roaster in your city. Visit the Web sites to get a sense of whether the place is run by coffee snobs who know their coffee (a good thing) or bored college kids (not such a good thing). In addition, this may sound odd, but in the hundreds of cities I have visited on business travel, the very best coffee shops have tended to have an unusually high number of tattoos and piercings (on the waitstaff, not the coffee). So look for a coffee place that smells like roasting coffee and is staffed with some really interesting-looking people.

A coffee shop that takes the time to select great-tasting coffee will often have at least one selection that will help you perform better and taste great, but the staff are unlikely to know which beans are the safest. If you ask, you will usually hear that none of the beans have mold toxins. But this is something no one can tell by looking because they are measured in parts per billion. (That's why I use lab tests!) You can reduce the amount of toxins in your coffee by insisting on single-origin coffee instead of accepting coffee blended from many locations. Coffee from Central America tends to be lower in toxins than coffee from other regions, but that is not always the case.

This can be time-consuming and doesn't guarantee results, so I simply travel with my own lab-tested beans, which I know I can trust to be virtually toxin-free and to give me a bigger and longer-lasting performance boost than any other coffee I've found. I believe that simplicity and laziness are virtues, so I don't waste time. This is not an issue of coffee snobbery. It simply matters that much to me to keep myself in a constant state of high performance!

BULLETPROOF INTERMITTENT FASTING

The idea of fasting for any length of time is a bit scary for all of us, and for good reason. This is because our Labrador brains are trained to think that the world is coming to an end when we stop eating, even for as few as 18 hours. But there are unquestionable benefits to short bouts of fasting, including a metabolic boost and sharper focus. "Intermittent fasting," which traditionally means eating all of your food within a shortened period of the day (usually 6 to 8 hours), has gained popularity among biohackers, weight lifters, and Paleo dieters because it is incredibly useful in aiding fat loss, preventing cancer, building muscle, and increasing resilience. This keeps you well fed and tells your body to simultaneously build muscle and burn fat

> I've had several GI issues since 2011, which led me to have to stop drinking green tea due to the caffeine, and at 36 years old I've never been a coffee drinker. However, based on my own biohacking journey, it sounded like I couldn't go wrong with Dave! My first cup of Bulletproof Coffee included the Brain Octane oil, which had an immediate mental alertness effect. The effect is so positive that it's all I need to hit the gym first thing in the morning feeling strong. **—Nick**

through some specific mechanisms I'll discuss in detail later. Intermittent fasting has been well researched and found to have a number of health benefits beyond weight loss and increased focus. Alternate-day fasting, one form of intermittent fasting, has been shown to prevent chronic disease, reduce triglycerides, and produce significant improvements in several markers such as LDL cholesterol in as little as 8 weeks.[16] Perhaps most importantly, intermittent fasting increases neuronal plasticity and neurogenesis, meaning it literally makes it easier for your brain to grow and evolve.[17]

There's just one problem with this fasting. Common intermittent-fasting protocols require you to skip breakfast and not eat lunch until after 2:00 p.m. That works great if you live in a cave, but if you're a parent holding down a full-time job like me, you'll probably find that your energy starts to decline right in the middle of your workday. Just when you want to be in a high-performance zone for work, your intermittent fast gets in the way. This problem led me to wonder if there was a way to get the benefits of intermittent fasting without scaring my Labrador brain into thinking it was the end of the species.

The other problem with intermittent fasting is that if you're significantly overweight it's even harder for you than it is for most people to skip meals and simply go about your day. When I experimented with intermittent fasting, I was often cranky and cold by midmorning, since it's common to have a lower body temperature while fasting. I looked for a way to hack this process. Since butter and Brain Octane Oil do not contain any protein, I knew my body would use them to quickly make ketones instead of

> I saw a friend I had not seen in 25 years, and he asked if I had ever
> heard of putting butter in coffee. He explained how it works and what it
> is supposed to do. This is a very intelligent guy, by the way, so I took his
> advice and ordered some beans and Brain Octane Oil from Bulletproof.
> At the time I weighed 288 pounds and entered a biggest-loser contest
> at my work. Needless to say, I crushed the competition. In 7 to 8 weeks,
> I lost about 70 pounds. The competition was supposed to last for
> 12 weeks, but I crushed everyone else so badly they all quit before
> the end. **—Jason Hood**

turning on protein or sugar digestion. I tried intermittent fasting while adding a cup of Bulletproof Coffee in the morning, and the results were amazing. I lost fat and built muscle even faster than I did with plain intermittent fasting and without ever feeling hungry or tired. The fat in my Bulletproof Coffee was so satiating that I could work straight through until lunchtime or even dinnertime with no distractions, but my body acted as if it was still fasting.

I call this new technique Bulletproof Intermittent Fasting, a simple hack that has allowed me to reap all the benefits of intermittent fasting with none of the negative side effects. It gives your body what it needs to perform well while totally ignoring food, tells your Labrador brain that all is well, and provides all the metabolic benefits of a fast. If you want to shed fat and improve your health as quickly as possible without slowing down, it's hard to beat Bulletproof Intermittent Fasting.

There are a few more reasons that Bulletproof Intermittent Fasting works better than just having no food at all during a plain intermittent-fasting plan. The first is that it triples down on a major physiological mechanism called mammalian target of rapamycin, or mTOR, which increases protein synthesis in your muscles and therefore helps build muscle. The more mTOR is suppressed, the stronger its action "springs back" and increases its muscle-building activity. Exercise suppresses mTOR in the moment, which is why you actually build muscle *after* you've finished working out and the mTOR bounces back, and not during the workout itself. The two other main ways of suppressing mTOR so that you'll build muscle later are intermittent fasting and coffee. After fasting, mTOR rises when you eat and builds more muscle. The same thing happens after drinking coffee. This is so powerful that you don't even need to hit on all three mTOR triggers (exercise, fasting, and coffee) to get staggering results. I did Bulletproof Intermittent Fasting regularly while eating more than 4,000 calories a day and never working out, and I still grew a six-pack.

The other reason Bulletproof Intermittent Fasting is so effective is that the Brain Octane Oil in Bulletproof Coffee helps you go into ketosis even if you've eaten some carbohydrates the day before. As I mentioned earlier, limiting carbs on the Bulletproof Diet is a powerful way to produce a state of metabolic ketosis, but Brain Octane Oil also helps the body get useful amounts of ketones very quickly without extreme carbohydrate restriction.

In addition to burning fat and helping you lose weight, ketosis increases your stamina. When your brain is running on ketones, you have more focus and don't experience the drops in energy level that are all too common on a high-carb diet because your blood sugar remains steady during ketosis. You switch your metabolism into fat-burning mode, which frees you from sudden energy crashes and brain fog. You'll likely feel the difference in your brain first, as even mild ketosis has an immediate cognitive impact.

To say I am in the best mental, physical, and spiritual state of my life would not be an exaggeration. I feel like a warrior. I can handle life's obstacles with a grin and energy. I have extreme focus and speed on completing any tasks, and my body has not been this lean and happy since I was a kid. My creativity and resourcefulness has also risen, my dreams grew, my life has changed, and I am absolutely excited to be journeying through it. I throw butter or ghee and Brain Octane Oil into any hot beverage I take. I do it all for me, but the look on people's faces who absolutely do not understand this life-changing concept is quite priceless. **—Gosia**

Ketogenic diets are nothing new, but Bulletproof Intermittent Fasting is a way to hack this established process to get the benefits of ketosis without the negative side effects or health risks. Staying in ketosis for too long can cause constipation, low body temperature, bad breath, adrenal fatigue, and even an accumulation of biogenic histamines in the bloodstream. By allowing you to dip in and out of ketosis through Bulletproof Intermittent Fasting, the Bulletproof Diet provides a mild state of ketosis and increases your overall metabolic health. This combination is just plain superior and will lead to a far-superior you.

The Bulletproof Intermittent Fasting feeding window is 6 hours long, giving you an 18-hour fast. This is the perfect length for an intermittent fast, but this part of the Bulletproof Diet isn't black-and-white. This is your opportunity to be your own biohacker and experiment to see what works best for you. If your fast is only 16 hours long, you'll still get some, but not all, of the benefits of an 18-hour fast. Once the fast shortens to less than 15 hours, you'll start to lose most of the benefits because it takes that long for the body to adapt to a fast, but you can play around with this window of 15 to 18 hours to see what gives you the best results and the most mojo. You can also take advantage of this window by eating dinner earlier the night before if you have a business lunch the next day. For example, if you have a business lunch at noon the next day and want to achieve a 15-hour fast, all you need to do is stop eating at 9:00 the night before.

For the first 2 weeks on the Bulletproof Diet, your breakfast will consist of Bulletproof Coffee with creamy, delicious butter and Brain Octane Oil (or coconut oil, which doesn't work nearly as well, as it's only 25 percent as powerful as Brain Octane Oil). Don't worry that this will leave you hungry. The fats will satiate you and tell your Labrador brain that all is well! Since your body does not really recognize fat as a meal when it is eaten without protein, carbs, or sugar, drinking Bulletproof Coffee in the morning instead of eating breakfast keeps you in fasting mode while satisfying your hunger and providing numerous benefits.

Once you're in maintenance mode, if you want to eat something in

> I have been eating Bulletproof for 2 months, and I have seen tremendous changes. My acne is gone, I have conquered food cravings, and I got straight A's for the first time ever because of my amazing focus from Bulletproof Coffee. Bulletproof has positively affected every aspect of my life, and I am beyond grateful. **—David**

addition to having Bulletproof Coffee in the morning, the best idea is to eat a combination of protein and fat, like poached eggs or smoked salmon and avocado. Eating just protein without any fats is better than eating fruits or other carbs, but this will still lead to some food cravings. Eating protein (or carbs like sugar) in the morning also kicks on your body's digestion process, which ends the "fast" you'd been in while you were asleep. Your liver will want to have a source of metabolic fuel to help break down the protein, so you'll get a food craving a couple hours later. Eating fat along with the protein will prevent this by giving your body extra energy to break down the protein into amino acids. Plus, it's more satisfying.

That said, if you are a woman, a heavily muscled athlete, or have a lot of weight to lose, you will likely benefit from having some protein with your Bulletproof Coffee in the morning for the first 60 days. This will help reset your leptin sensitivity.[18] For these people, I recommend blending collagen protein from grass-fed cows right into your Bulletproof Coffee. It's flavorless and invisible, and it's good for your connective tissue, too. I do this a few times a week.

EAT CARBS FOR DESSERT, NOT BREAKFAST

Eating carbs in the morning will set you up for an energy spike and crash along with food cravings throughout the entire day. If you decide to test this for yourself, it will be blindingly obvious. Try having just Bulletproof Coffee instead of your usual breakfast and see how long it takes you to want food.

For most people, it turns off the desire for food for at least 5 to 6 hours. Then try having protein with your Bulletproof Coffee for breakfast. You'll probably be full for approximately 4 to 5 hours—not as long as if you'd had a pure-fat breakfast. Next, try eating a high-protein, low-fat breakfast with or without vegetables. You'll be satisfied, but for an even shorter amount of time. Finally, eat a bagel with low-fat spread or a bowl of cereal with fat-free milk for breakfast. It will only take about 2 to 3 hours until you have an intense desire for more food—most likely something like a doughnut. Oatmeal without fat will "stick to your ribs" a bit longer than a bagel, but not nearly as long as protein or fat.

Eating carbs for breakfast not only leaves you hungry, but also takes you out of ketosis, which you should be in at least some of the time in order to keep your brain running at full speed. For all of these reasons, some diets famously recommended eating virtually no carbs at all, but as you read earlier, this sets you up for another host of problems.

One reason the time of day you eat your carbs is so important is that you want to avoid continually feeding the bad bacteria in your gut throughout the day. As you read earlier, hungry bacteria make FIAF, which causes you to burn fat. When gut bacteria are fed sugar or starch, they stop producing FIAF and you start storing fat.[19] Feeding your gut bacteria starch and sugar all day long is a terrible idea because it will cause your body to

I started off trying Bulletproof Coffee with garbage coffee and garbage butter, but when I took the time to try out the real thing it was a totally different experience. My brain worked better, and I love how I think and reason while running on fats. When studying for the MCAT for 6 months, I drank Bulletproof Coffee every morning. On the day of the test, I walked in with a big thermos of Bulletproof Coffee and a lot of confidence. I knew that I would have the mental energy to attack the test. While Bulletproof Coffee wasn't the only thing that led to my success on the MCAT—I also hacked my sleep, hit the books like it was my job, and got my diet in check—but it definitely was a major building block of my overall test-taking strategy. —**Eugene**

> By incorporating healthy fats from grass-fed butter and Brain Octane Oil into my Upgraded Coffee, I have healthy energy that lasts all day. I'm keeping my joints and ligaments healthy by adding grass-fed collagen into the mix, and including grass-fed whey to make sure I'm getting the best protein to keep muscle recovery a top priority! I recommend the Bulletproof protocols to anyone trying to up their game in any facet of their life! **—Samuel Shaw, professional wrestler with TNA Impact Wrestling**

store fat instead of burning it. This is why bacteria-rich yogurt isn't a great breakfast, either.

As a biohacker, I had to test this out. For 1 week, I added Jerusalem artichoke extract, a powerful source of prebiotic fiber that gut bacteria love, to my Bulletproof Coffee. I swallowed a commonly sold stomach-acid-resistant probiotic capsule at the same time. The results? I gained 10 pounds in a week and my pants didn't fit. It was gross. I don't own "fat pants" anymore, and I had no intention of buying them! It took 7 days to lose those 10 pounds using normal Bulletproof techniques. This taught me that gut bacteria should be fed during specific times of the day to promote FIAF production and avoid unnecessary weight gain.

The Bulletproof solution is to eat a modest amount of Bulletproof carbs (about 30 grams, plus vegetables), but only with your evening meal or soon after. Once or twice a week, eat 100 to 150 grams. The exact amount depends on your hunger, your stress levels, and how fast you want to lose weight. (Eating fewer carbs nightly brings faster weight loss.) There are a few reasons it's important to eat your carbs at night. The first is that your body uses starch and sugar to make serotonin, a neurotransmitter that relaxes you and helps you sleep. If carbs are going to make you relaxed and cause your energy level to drop, you might as well time this for when you want to go to sleep instead of when you need to perform and focus. It's also helpful to be asleep by the time your Labrador brain feels that energy crash and begins demanding more sugar. Finally, the extra blood sugar you get from eating carbs at night will help your brain do the work it needs to do while you're sleeping. This will dramatically improve your quality of sleep while allowing your body to produce moderate levels of ketones and providing raw materials to form tears and mucus. Tears and mucus are made from carbohydrates, and it's metabolically difficult for some people to make enough tears by converting protein to glucose.

This is my primary way of achieving all of the low-carb benefits without the established problems that come from long-term low-carb dieting. The proper timing of carbs is one way the Bulletproof Diet works like it does. Any other long-term, high-fat, moderate-protein, low-carb diet simply won't allow you to achieve the same results.

BULLETPROOF PROTEIN FASTING

Through my antiaging nonprofit work, I discovered some interesting information about the body's natural cleaning process, called autophagy, which recycles the junk in your cells and turns it into energy. This is the cellular equivalent of burning your trash to stay warm. Over time, cells accumulate dead organelles, damaged proteins, and oxidized particles that interfere with cell function and accelerate aging. Autophagy is the body's method of clearing out this clutter, meaning it helps keep you young. Clearly, autophagy is something you want your cells to do well in order to look, feel, and perform your best.

> For several long years, I counted calories, monitored nutrient intake, clocked in several hours a week doing cardio, and became vegan. Yet there was no progress. I felt amazing with tons of vegetables in my body, but I developed issues digesting my legumes and had insatiable cravings for carbs. The worst part is I never felt full and never kept weight off. I started to accept the fact I would just never have control of my body, and that this was simply my own personal "optimal" state. It wasn't until I stumbled upon Bulletproof Coffee (and eventually the Bulletproof Diet) that I realized what "optimal" truly meant. **—Arielle**

Autophagy is required to maintain muscle mass, and it inhibits muscle breakdown in adults.[20] Since I was interested in staying younger and building muscle by spending less time working out (and who isn't?), I was determined to hack autophagy. I started by looking at the two main signals for the body to turn on autophagy. The first is fasting. I realized that this was one of the reasons I was experiencing such amazing results with Bulletproof Intermittent Fasting, but through my research I found there was an even better way to turn on autophagy, and that's by occasionally limiting protein consumption. When you do this, you force your cells to find every possible way to recycle proteins. In their search, they bind and excrete toxins that were lurking in your cell's cytoplasm, the gel-like substance enclosed within the cell membrane. It's like taking your car to the car wash and having it deep cleaned.

Studies have shown a number of additional benefits to being protein deficient that are similar to the benefits of fasting. The first is that protein deficiency lowers insulin and mTOR. Remember, stomping down mTOR so its secretion can spring back up is key to building muscle. The problem was, I had spent almost a year as a raw vegan, which automatically limited protein, and found that it caused me many health problems. In fact, being chronically protein deficient is awful for your brain and your body. The trick was to come up with a way to become *temporarily* protein deficient.

The simplest way to do this is to do a traditional fast and eat nothing for 24 hours or longer. I decided to experiment with this and do it right. In 2008, I arranged to be dropped off about 20 miles outside of Sedona, Arizona, in a national forest where there was a little-known cave. I brought a sleeping bag, water, a knife, and a cell phone in case of emergencies. I meditated there for 4 days and lost about 15 pounds. Since I was eating nothing at all, there's no doubt I was benefiting from autophagy, but I was also benefiting from the fact that fasting caused my gut bacteria to secrete FIAF so I could burn fat. (Not to mention the fact that I was eating no calories at all.)

When I returned to civilization, I wanted to experience the benefits of autophagy without all the fuss, but eating nothing for 24 or 48 hours is inconvenient if you have a job or friends. The hack for this is Bulletproof Protein Fasting. On 1 day per week, I started limiting my protein to no more than 25 grams. As I experimented with different amounts, a good friend and fellow biohacker named Josh Whiton told me to aim for 15 grams or less instead of 25 and to be more rigorous in my counting. I hadn't realized that most foods that say they have zero grams of protein per serving on the Nutrition Facts label actually do have some protein that adds up when eaten in quantity. Coconut cream is a good example. The label says it has no protein *in a serving size of 2 tablespoons.* But when I was sipping a delicious quarter cup of the stuff on a protein-fasting day, I was getting a full gram of sneaky protein. Indeed, when I switched to a strict 15 grams a day, I felt a huge difference and had a visible reduction in my abdominal inflammation and muffin top. (No, I don't walk around looking like a fashion model every day. Muffin top happens to the best of us!)

Now, on the 1 day a week I'm Bulletproof Protein Fasting, I basically eat a vegetarian diet of Bulletproof foods with less than 15 grams of protein, including some Bulletproof carbs and tons of fat. Later in the book, I'll provide you with specific meal plans you can follow on your protein-fasting day. Keep in mind this is not a cheat day. Do not give yourself permission to hit up all of your local fast-food joints and then eat an entire cake! Bulletproof Protein Fasting is simply a great way to get an even better reduction in inflammation and superior Bulletproof results.

Like Bulletproof Intermittent Fasting, Bulletproof Protein Fasting is not an all-or-nothing deal. If you find that a full day of protein fasting is causing muscle loss or some other unwanted side effects, cut back so that instead of going a whole day without protein, you're skipping protein at several meals in a row. You can also play around with the total amount of protein you're eating on the day of your Bulletproof Protein Fast. This is another great opportunity to be your own biohacker in order to get optimum results. I tried eating only protein at dinner, but didn't get much of the slimming effect, so I either do it right—for a full day at 15 grams of protein or less—or I just don't do it.

WHEN TO EAT

The Simple Bulletproof Diet

Designed to reduce body fat, enhance mental performance,
and prevent disease while leaving you satisfied and energized.

Eat when you're hungry, stop when you're satiated, and try not to snack. Target 50–70% of calories
from healthy fats, 20% from protein, 20% vegetables, and 5% fruit or starch. For optimal results,
follow the dark portion of the diet and limit fruit or starch consumption to 1–2 servings per day in
the evenings to avoid high triglycerides.

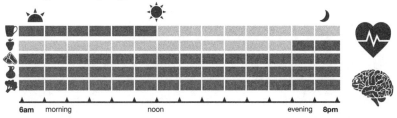

Bulletproof Intermittent Fasting for Fat Loss and Focus

A biohack that makes it possible to lose fat, while increasing
mental focus and energy, without cravings.

You start by consuming a cup of Bulletproof Coffee in the morning. The healthy fats give you a
stable current of energy, and the ultra low-toxin Bulletproof Coffee beans optimize brain function
and fat loss. For optimal results, follow the top portion of the diet in conjunction with this protocol.

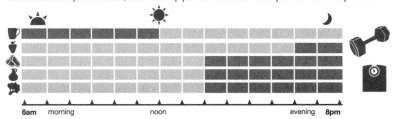

Bulletproof Protein Fasting

A biohack used occasionally to get a greater reduction
in inflammation.

About 1–2 times a week, limit your protein intake to 15–25g to help cleanse your inner cells
without muscle loss. To keep you full and energized, consume a cup of Bulletproof Coffee in the
morning and have high fats and moderate carbs throughout the day. For optimal results, follow
the top portion of the diet and limit carbohydrates to the afternoon and evening.

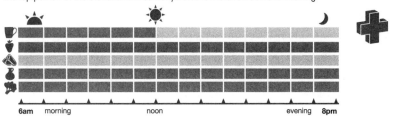

Download your free color copy at http://bulletproof.com/roadmap.

CHAPTER

5

SLEEP BETTER AND BOOST YOUR ENERGY

Most people have horrible sleep fitness. They waste time falling asleep and then spend hours in a light sleep state that doesn't have the same body- and brain-boosting benefits of deep and REM sleep. This used to be me. I'd spend an hour trying to fall asleep because my brain wouldn't stop rehashing the day's events or dwelling on what was coming up the next day. I woke up every morning still feeling groggy.

Sleep also seemed like a waste of precious time. There was always something more interesting to do. Throughout my life I've tried several different sleep experiments because I wanted to spend more time experiencing life and less time sleeping. Back in high school, I slept 3 to 4 hours at night (from 3:00 to 6:00 a.m.) and then arrived at school so exhausted that I was famous for taking a nap in almost every class. That meant an additional 1½ hours of sleep broken into 15-minute naps spread across six periods.

(Since I was ranked second in my class, my teachers let me get away with this.) On Fridays and Saturdays, I'd sleep for 10 to 12 hours a night, putting my weekly average at between 6.5 and 7.3 hours of sleep per night. This was not efficient, nor did it improve my health, and there's evidence that people under the age of 20 need extra sleep. I also found that I had to rely on soda to remain alert when I wasn't sleeping in class. In college, my schedule was more flexible and I decided to follow my natural circadian rhythm. I found that when class schedules allowed, I naturally stayed up until 6:00 a.m. and then slept until 11:00 a.m. or noon. This method didn't really save a lot of time and didn't seem to help with alertness, either.

While starting my career, I decided to complete two semesters of computer information systems classes in a single semester. I slept 2 to 3 hours per night (from 5:00 to 7:00) and then drove to school barely awake before downing 40 to 60 ounces of coffee and starting a day of classes. I felt awesome until crashing 3 hours later and then struggling to make it through the rest of the day. I worked out with weights several times a week in an effort to gain more energy. In retrospect, I realize that I gave myself adrenal fatigue and probably hurt my thyroid function with this experiment because the intense workouts and so little sleep were putting so much stress on my body. Then I read about polyphasic sleep, which involves sleeping for 20 minutes at a time every 4 hours. I tried it briefly a year or two later, but the massive inconvenience and rigidity of the schedule in no way made up for the few hours of sleep it saved.

All these years of experimenting with sleep helped me learn more about sleep quality, which is determined by how fast you fall asleep and how much time you spend in REM and delta (deep, restorative) sleep. Through a combination of self-experimenting and biohacking, I've finally learned how to optimize my sleep quality and recovery, and this has allowed me to have more experiences than most people my age. I've been fortunate enough to run strategy for two different billion-dollar companies, have three of my companies acquired, work for a venture capital firm, teach for 5 years at the University of California, advise dozens of startups, run an antiaging nonprofit, become host of a nationally syndicated radio show, and start the Bulletproof Executive and number one–ranked iTunes podcast with information that's reached millions. But life isn't just professional accomplishments. It's personal. I also spend lots of time with my lovely wife, Lana, and our two young kids. In the last 3 years, I've found extra time to go through several weeklong 40 Years of Zen programs to teach my brain new abilities that normally take years of meditation. This is an intense program I use with executive coaching clients to quickly control stress and increase performance, and it requires you to be connected to a neurofeedback (electroencephalogram) machine for a week, focused entirely on making your brain do what an advanced Zen master's brain does.

One of the reasons I've been able to do all this is because I taught myself to sleep less than most people. Based on Americans' average sleep time, over the first half of my life, I've had roughly an extra 8 years to live without being tired all the time. It really is possible to reap all the benefits of sleep in less time. You can train your brain to sleep better, and healthy people need less sleep in the first place because they recover faster.

Sleep is an important part of the Bulletproof Diet because there is actually a direct link between your diet and your sleep. What you eat directly affects how well you sleep, and the quality of your sleep also has a dramatic impact on your weight loss (or gain) and your performance. Getting high-quality sleep is one of the most important variables in improving your brain function, longevity, and performance in all aspects of life. Life is too short to wake up tired!

Most people still equate good sleep with getting 8 consecutive hours, but a University of California at San Diego paper on sleep research and aging reviewed data from 1.1 million people and determined that there is no statistical reason to sleep longer than 6½ hours per night. In fact, the people who slept 6½ hours a night lived longer than the ones who slept 8 hours.[1] No, this doesn't mean that sleeping for 8 hours a night will kill you, but it might mean that if it takes 9 or 10 hours of sleep for you to feel human you're less healthy than someone who feels great after only 6½ hours. In short, the healthier and more Bulletproof you are, the less sleep you might need. This is not a license to starve yourself of sleep, but just as more protein is not always better, more sleep is not always better, either. It's about getting the right quality and the right amount for you!

Ultimately, the quality of your sleep is much more important than the quantity, and getting good-quality sleep is important, indeed. Lack of good sleep can make you fat, give you cancer and heart disease, and substantially increase your risk of dying, while quality sleep has a slew of major benefits for your mind and body. One good night of sleep can improve "motor speed without loss of accuracy" in executing a new motor skill by 20 percent compared to not sleeping,[2] while getting quality sleep increases your ability to gain new insight into cognitive tasks by 50 percent.[3] Meanwhile, good sleep promotes skin health and a youthful appearance,[4] controls optimal insulin secretion,[5] encourages healthy cell division,[6] and increases athletic performance.[7]

So how do you improve the quality of your sleep? The trick is to upgrade your metabolism with the Bulletproof Diet and then hack your sleep so you can sleep even better. Now it is possible to literally gain more hours in the day while preserving and often even boosting your health, mental function, and energy. Unhacked sleep takes forever—about 34 percent of your life if you sleep as much as your body will let you without an alarm clock waking you up (or two young kids, in my case). If you Bulletproof your sleep and cut it down to only 20 percent of your life, you will still sleep about 5 hours a night. Assuming you live to 80, cutting

> I have a very strict diet, which does not include gluten, dairy, aspartame, etc. I take lots of supplements, and I have a stash (a rather large one) of incandescent bulbs! I am so glad that my friend turned me on to you. It is so wonderful to hear someone preaching this message. —**Julie**

sleep to 5 hours a night is like gaining an additional 16 years of waking life. Think about what you would do with all that extra time. You could get five master's degrees, start another career, enjoy a lot more sex, play with your kids, or you could just play bingo. It's your time. Own it.

Bulletproofing your sleep doesn't mean that you *have* to sleep for less than 6 hours a night. In fact, at the time I'm writing this, my average night's sleep over the last 456 days is exactly 6 hours and 1 minute according to one of the two sleep-tracking systems I use (although I did go for 2 years on less than 5 hours per night). Even if you already sleep 8 or more hours a night and plan to continue that, you will greatly benefit from improving the quality of your sleep. But when you're practicing the Bulletproof Diet in combination with these sleep-efficiency hacks, you can almost always sleep less without suffering the negative effects of lost sleep. If you're obese or suffering from chronic illness, deal with that before you hack your sleep!

If you can't sleep, there are three main reasons for it—either you're not tired, you're distracted, or you have a biological problem (a "hardware problem" in hacker speak) such as sleep apnea or hormone irregularities that needs medical attention. Well, the first two of these possible issues are pretty easy to control. If you're living in a state of high performance, sleep should be a conscious act, not something that just happens. You have the power to do specific things to make sure you're tired when you decide to go to sleep. This includes eating the right foods at the right times, taking supplements and/or drugs, and using technology.

DIET HACKS FOR BETTER SLEEP

In 2012, researchers identified a new maintenance system called the glymphatic system, which uses the cells' mitochondria to remove cellular waste from the brain.[8] They noted that this system is particularly active during sleep. In other words, as you sleep your brain cells' mitochondria remove cellular waste. If you improve your mitochondrial function during sleep, you'll turbocharge your brain's maintenance system and get more cleanup done in fewer hours of sleep.

Some core practices on the Bulletproof Diet improve mitochondrial function. In 2013, another team of researchers learned that autophagy is required for healthy brain cell mitochondria.[9] Remember what increases autophagy? That's right—Bulletproof Intermittent Fasting and Protein Fasting. The very shortest-chain MCT oil also provides ketones, which act as fuel for the mitochondria. If you follow the Bulletproof Diet, you're already upgrading your brain's ability to drain waste as you sleep.

This means that by itself, following the Bulletproof Diet will help most people get better quality sleep, but sometimes we can all use a little boost. As someone who wants to perform your best, you want to do everything possible to increase cellular energy in the brain while you sleep. Formula 1 race car mechanics are obsessive about how they maintain and fuel their high-performance machines. Your brain is the highest-performing machine in your body. Increasing its efficiency pays dividends during waking hours and even more so during sleep.

There are several ways beyond the basic Bulletproof Diet to use your diet to improve your sleep, but certain dietary sleep hacks work better for some people than others. This is highly variable, so customize your own ultimate sleep plan by taking this opportunity to be your own biohacker to find out which of these sleep hacks works best for you. Don't try all of the dietary sleep hacks at once because they work in different ways and can counteract each other. Try them out one at a time and see which ones supercharge your sleep.

FILL UP WITH FAT AT DINNER

This hack works for almost everyone and is an inherent part of the Bulletproof Diet. Fat is a long-burning fuel for your mind and body, and filling up with clean fats at dinner gives you a steady stream of energy. Grass-fed butter, animal fat, and coconut oil are all good choices, but extra-concentrated MCT oil is my personal favorite. The shortest-length

> As a courtroom lawyer that needs to be focused and on his toes, the Bulletproof Diet gives me the edge I need to win! By eliminating foods that are high in toxins and eating a ton of good fat found in grass-fed butter and Brain Octane Oil, the Bulletproof Diet helps me function at high levels during high stress and with little sleep. It's my secret weapon during trial! —**William E. Johnson, West Palm Beach, Florida**

fats of MCT oil are converted into ketones that are immediately used as fuel for your brain, and MCT oil also helps you burn body fat while you sleep. I've noticed that I think faster and more clearly the next morning if I have 1 to 2 tablespoons of Brain Octane Oil the night before with dinner or even right before bed. Try drinking the No-Coffee Vanilla Latte (see page 254), which contains Brain Octane Oil, as a Bulletproof nightcap. Like Bul- letproof Coffee, this drink will not take you out of the fasting state with- out added protein.

Caution: If you're not used to any Brain Octane Oil at all, start slowly and be sure to mix it into something (as in the Vanilla Latte) so it is gentler on your stomach. As I mentioned earlier, too much Brain Octane Oil can cause the runs, which will definitely prevent you from sleeping well!

FUEL WITH LOW-MERCURY FISH (OR KRILL) OIL

DHA, an omega-3 fatty acid, has a lot of benefits, such as protecting against the negative effects of fructose on brain function, improving mood and reducing anxiety and depression, improving insulin sensitivity, and increasing muscle growth. Studies have shown that fish oil, which contains DHA, aids in the secretion of serotonin, a neurotransmitter that promotes feelings of wellness and lowers levels of stress hormones that can interfere with sleep.[10]

I've experimented with various kinds of fish oil and pretty much every other omega-3 supplement you can think of, and I've found that krill oil gives me the best sleep. In fact, it's the only one that has made a noticeable impact. I recommend consuming 1 gram of fish or krill oil either with dinner or at bedtime. Avoid flaxseed oil and hemp-seed oil because they are high in omega-6s and low in omega-3s and are not Bulletproof foods.

PRIME WITH PROTEIN

Our bodies use protein for muscle repair and immune function. The muscle repair happens at night during deep sleep, so you want to make sure your body has all the raw materials it needs at night to heal and grow new tissue. The problem is that most forms of protein are not well digested before bed. A lot of protein powders and even most sources of animal protein take a lot of work to digest and can leave you with a heavy feeling during the night. The resources that are used to digest these proteins would also be better used fueling your brain. Too much protein also raises an alertness chemical in the brain called orexin, which can disrupt your sleep. The solution I recommend is taking 1 to 2 tablespoons of hydrolyzed grass-fed collagen peptide before bed. Hydrolyzing the proteins makes them more digestible so they don't cause the problems listed above. You can mix this right into your No-Coffee Vanilla Latte and benefit from two sleep hacks at once, as the Brain Octane Oil in the latte will give your body the extra energy it needs to break down the protein.

ENJOY THE POWER OF WHEY PROTEIN

This is another option that can be taken instead of (not in addition to) collagen protein. Grass-fed, undenatured whey protein concentrate is easy to digest, is full of essential amino acids for repairing your body tissue, and contains bioactive milk peptides (BMPs). BMPs are one of the most promising new supplements for improving sleep and reducing stress. They are actually derived from whey protein, but they are a lot more expensive after processing, so you might as well eat them from the source.

These proteins are most effective in their undenatured form. Heating and pressurizing them reduces their effects, which is why I always prefer to get BMPs from cold processed whey protein concentrate rather than in pill form. The other benefit of this form of whey protein is that it raises your liver's glutathione levels. Glutathione helps your liver remove toxins that interfere with sleep. If it works for you, try taking 1 to 2 tablespoons of super-high-quality grass-fed, low-temperature-processed whey at night in your No-Coffee Vanilla Latte.

TRY RAW HONEY

This is a powerful sleep hack that you should try on its own, not in combination with the protein supplements listed above. Your brain uses a lot of energy while you're sleeping. One efficient form of brain energy comes from the sugar that is stored in your liver, called liver glycogen. Your brain taps your liver glycogen before hitting the stored sugar in your muscles (muscle glycogen), so having a little carbohydrate before bed can help your brain function better at night. Raw honey is used preferentially to the stock of liver glycogen, so it is used first for brain function. Raw honey is 22 percent better at making liver glycogen than the processed conventional stuff you're likely to find at most grocery stores that has the pollen filtered out.[11] Taking a small amount of honey by itself before bed will raise blood glucose while you sleep, putting you in a deeper sleep faster.

As I mentioned earlier, the late Seth Roberts discussed this sleep hack with me as he was developing his self-experiments on the effect of carefully timed carbohydrates before sleep. He also found, as I did, that honey improved his sleep, but he found it also improved his strength and resilience, too.[12] He used himself as a guinea pig to gather excruciating levels of data validating that it worked for him, and Nathaniel Altman's book *The Honey Prescription* also reveals these strengthening powers of honey. This trick really can help you get more deep sleep, especially when you're doing Bulletproof Intermittent Fasting. At first I assumed the honey

I had sleeping problems for over 20 years and now I can sleep! I'm losing weight faster than I can believe and it feels amazing. The other people I know on the Bulletproof Diet can say the same and are excited that their health is finally taking shape. **—Michelle** would throw me out of fat-burning mode, but as long as I took Brain Octane Oil with the honey, I produced enough ketones to stay in mild fat-burning mode. The shortest length MCT, C8, does produce ketones even in the presence of carbohydrates, so you can stay in a mild state of ketosis while benefiting from this sleep hack.

SUPPLEMENT YOUR SLEEP

For some people, using the food hacks above is enough to supercharge their sleep, but some will need even more help from supplements. These are some of the best ones for taking your sleep to the next level so you can feel great and thrive on fewer hours a night of higher-quality sleep. I take most of these on most nights and track how effective they are by using a sleep-tracking app on my phone. Always check your supplements to verify they are compatible with medications you may be taking.

Note: I'm specifically avoiding many herbs because the common ones recommended for sleep (like valerian root) have always left me feeling groggy in the morning. Who wants to go to sleep fast only to then waste the entire morning in a fog?

MAGNESIUM

Almost everyone is short on magnesium, and you should be taking it anyway if you want to live a long life. (I'll talk about this more in Chapter 7.) Try taking 600 to 800 mg a day, but be careful because too much magnesium can gives you "disaster pants" (which doesn't help you sleep). The best forms are the "-ates," including malate, citrate, aspartate, and others. Since it is relaxing, most people benefit from taking magnesium in the evening.

POTASSIUM

This is synergistic with magnesium, and for most people with nighttime leg cramps, the combination will help. My preferred forms are citrate and potassium bicarbonate, which is harder to find. Potassium keeps the heart

HUMAN GROWTH HORMONE

During sleep, your body naturally secretes human growth hormone (HGH), which maintains your organs and tissues. As you age, the amount of HGH that your body secretes naturally decreases. This decline in HGH is correlated with many of the effects of aging. If you want to remain youthful, full of energy, and resilient, you should do everything in your power to keep your HGH levels high. Antiaging physicians and movie stars use it as an off-label prescription treatment for aging (which the FDA does not approve at this time), but you can use many of the supplements in this chapter to naturally cause your body to secrete more.

beating rhythmically, so too much potassium can alter your heartbeat—do not megadose. I take 400 mg of potassium citrate at bedtime. Start with 100 to 200 mg and work your way up from there if you feel you need more.

L-THEANINE

This is an amino acid found in green tea that is known to reduce stress. Its chemical structure resembles glutamic acid, which interferes with the function of glutamate. As you read earlier, glutamate is an excitatory neurotransmitter, and L-theanine reduces that excitatory effect and causes relaxation. I use 100 mg of Suntheanine, a specific form of L-theanine, at night.

GABA

This is an inhibitory neurotransmitter, what your brain uses to shut itself down. It will dramatically calm you when taken without any protein, so don't combine this one with the protein supplement recommendations above. Start with 500 mg. I used to swear by this, but I don't need it to go to sleep anymore now that I hacked my brain at 40 Years of Zen. Yet, there is evidence that 2,500 mg of GABA before bed will raise human growth hormone moderately, so I take that much most nights for antiaging purposes. While it's best for most of us to take GABA at night to induce sleep, I've also recommended it to stressed-out executives for use during the day when they were really tweaking and it calmed them down considerably.

PHENYL-GABA (PHENIBUT)

Phenibut is a supplement that is a derivative of GABA, but much stronger. It was discovered in Russia and is considered a nootropic (substance that helps your brain work better) because it can help with focus and then help to cause profound sleep. Unfortunately, phenibut does not absorb well past the gut and blood-brain barriers, although it does so more easily when it is packaged in a molecule that crosses through membranes, such as a liposomal delivery system. Look for liposomes on the label. As an added reason to consider it when you really want good sleep, Russian researchers found that phenibut protected against the psychological side effects of chronic stress in mice.

This is a very powerful sleep hack, one of my favorites, but keep your dose to less than 600 mg, and don't use it every day or it will stop working. There are reports of people abusing it by taking high doses for long periods of time and becoming dependent on it.[13] This is a very powerful sleep hack, but it doesn't mix with alcohol or some other medications.

ORNITHINE

This relaxing amino acid helps your body eliminate ammonia in the gut, as excess ammonia causes feelings of stress.[14] Ammonia is a cellular toxin, and eliminating it can improve your long- and short-term memories. Some people sleep much better with ornithine, and it may improve human growth hormone levels, too.[15] I take a mixture of arginine and ornithine at night for growth hormone release. Since digesting protein produces ammonia in the gut, ornithine may be particularly helpful if you're eating toward the higher recommended protein amounts on the Bulletproof Diet. Try taking from 500 to 1,000 mg at bedtime.

L-TRYPTOPHAN

In the late 1980s, one of the top manufacturers of L-tryptophan made a manufacturing error that possibly contaminated the supplement and linked L-tryptophan to a rare neurological condition called eosinophilia-myalgia syndrome. Mass hysteria resulted, even though properly produced L-tryptophan caused no issues, and all L-tryptophan was taken off the market. It's again available over the counter, and I recommend this powerful stuff, especially when it's taken with GABA. However, excessive amounts of L-tryptophan from food or supplements can be inflammatory, so don't overdo this one. Start with 500 mg a night. Many people associate L-tryptophan with Thanksgiving dinner, and while there may be a little bit of it in your turkey, eating it along with the amino acids in the protein make it unlikely that you'll feel an effect.

MELATONIN

This is a potent hormone and antioxidant that your body is supposed to produce on its own if you get real darkness and enough sleep. Since you probably get neither, there is an open debate around whether you should supplement every day and risk further depressing your natural melatonin production or just do it occasionally. Your body naturally regulates its production of hormones based on how much of those hormones are present in the body, so if you supplement with melatonin your body will naturally make less. Antiaging researchers generally believe that you should maintain your body's natural hormone production as much as possible, so I only use it one or two nights a week when I want power sleep, or when traveling. Unfortunately, most melatonin supplements are too strong. I recommend 300 to 500 mcg for men and 300 mcg for women, but the common dosage you can buy is 3 mg (3,000 mcg). In the short term for jet lag, you can safely use 1 to 3 mg.

VITAMIN D

Some sleep disorders are tied to vitamin D deficiency, which hurts the amount of sleep you get, the quality of your sleep, and your mood upon waking up. Unfortunately, many of us have a vitamin D deficiency because of the way we live—we work inside, wear clothes, and use sunscreen. These are all realities of modern life, and they all take away from our inherent vitamin D synthesis.

Contrary to what your mom may have told you, your body does not literally "soak up" vitamin D from the sun. Instead, the interaction between ultraviolet B light waves and a cholesterol derivative in the skin causes D to be synthesized in the body. While many of us wish we could quit our jobs and move to the Bahamas to get the rays we need, that is not realistic for most of us. Eating foods rich in vitamin D and supplementing with D_3 is necessary to maintain adequate D levels, but how much you take and when you take it are important variables.

According to the Vitamin D Council, 1,000 IU per 25 pounds of body weight are recommended each day, although using a blood test is the best way to determine your ideal dose. It's important not to take too much vitamin D for long periods of time, as excess amounts can cause head-aches and inflammation. Short-term megadoses are quite safe. A healthy human utilizes about 3,000 to 10,000 IU of vitamin D per day. These amounts are adjusted according to your age, weight, absorption of vitamin D through the layers of the skin, skin color, and normal sun exposure. The US government's tolerable upper limit (UL) for vitamin D is set at 4,000 IU per day for adults. Other experts disagree; many state it should be 5,000 to 10,000 IU. I recommend checking your blood level every 6 months.

Vitamin D is inversely related to your sleep hormone melatonin, so it makes sense that taking it at night disrupts your sleep. I've noticed this effect personally, and find that taking vitamin D in the morning is best for quality sleep at night. Quantified Self pioneer Seth Roberts docu-mented the same results.

ACTIVATED COCONUT CHARCOAL

Studies have found a connection between sleep deficits and bad gut bac-teria in animals.[16] Eating the Bulletproof Diet is a great way to optimize your gut bacteria, but sometimes you need a little extra help. Activated coconut charcoal acts like a vacuum cleaner by adsorbing or attaching to the toxins in your digestive tract before they can reach your brain and cause inflammation. This is especially useful if you are feeling unexplained anxiety at bedtime or after consuming antinutrients or alcohol. Don't mix this with pharmaceuticals or other protein-containing substances, as it will mop them up, too. Too much activated coconut charcoal can cause the opposite of "disaster pants," constipation. Start with 1 or 2 capsules and reduce the amount if you have this complication.

GLUTATHIONE

Glutathione is one of the most powerful antioxidants and detoxifiers your body makes. It's essential for removing toxins, protecting fats from oxidation, and assisting in immune system and brain function. The brain and liver have the highest concentrations of glutathione. Many people have lower-than-optimal glutathione levels due to stress, infections, poor diet, and other problems. If you're low on glutathione, your body can easily get overwhelmed by toxins and inflammation. While activated coconut charcoal targets toxins in your gut, an orally absorbable form of glutathione helps your liver remove toxins that are already in your bloodstream and other tissues. This means you get a more complete detox and even more

I've learned to cherish a good night's sleep. Sleeplessness can suck. It can especially suck when you have a new job with a lot to learn, when your eyes burn, when you get home exhausted, when it takes hours to fall asleep and yet you still wake up at the crack of dawn against your will, and still tired. Dave changed this for me in an evening, beginning with a Bulletproof dinner for me and a joint shopping trip for sleep-hacking nutrients at Whole Foods. The best part? He labeled each bottle with how much to take and when. He made it easy for me. I'd resigned myself to chronic exhaustion, and it made a difference to my work and to my relationship to learn what my body needed to sleep through the night and wake in the morning feeling rested and game. **—Gayle Karen Young, chief cultural and talent officer, Wikimedia Foundation** profound improvements in sleep quality[17]—in fact a lack of sleep is shown to decrease glutathione levels in the brain.[18]

Glutathione doesn't normally work when you take it orally because your body digests it before you can use it. I've used IV glutathione for more than a decade to detox, but this means going to the doctor's office and is expensive. When I travel I now take oral glutathione that has been encapsulated in MCT-based lipids along with lactoferrin to allow it to flow through the lining of the gut and dramatically raise my blood level of glutathione. This is the same technique used in advanced pharmaceutical delivery systems, but here it's used to more efficiently bring a natural substance into the body. On a recent trip to New York, I forgot to pack my glutathione and came down with laryngitis. A local antiaging physician kindly offered to administer an IV dose of 1.2 g, which helped the laryngitis resolve in 12 hours. I was able to give a talk about autism the next day. Without the glutathione, I would have had to whisper my speech.

ACTIVE PQQ

As you read earlier in this chapter, your cells' mitochondria play a key role in your brain's glymphatic detox system. The most impactful supplement I've tried for cranking up mitochondria is a unique active form of a cousin of the antioxidant coenzyme Q_{10} called pyrroloquinoline quinone, or PQQ for short. This is an up-and-coming supplement that has been shown in studies to make mitochondria work better[19] and help grow new ones.[20] Unfortunately, PQQ comes as a disodium salt, which had no discernable impact on my sleep even after taking a high oral dose of 30 mg per day for 2 years. However, the active form of PQQ, ActivePQQ, has had a profound impact on my sleep efficiency with only 10 mg. The first time I took it, I needed an hour less sleep to feel amazing.

TECH TIPS FOR BETTER SLEEP

The tools that follow are not part of the standard Bulletproof Diet, but they are powerful upgrades that you can use to improve your quality of sleep even more. This may be over the top for some people, but if you're relentlessly pursuing a perfect night's sleep (or just a tech geek like me), you'll love experimenting with some really effective toys to help supercharge your sleep. If you are under a lot of stress or if you travel frequently across time zones, some of these tools will give you a truly unfair advantage.

TRACK YOUR SLEEP QUALITY

My favorite smartphone sleep app, Sleep Cycle, simply requires you to put your phone on your mattress under your bottom sheet and set the alarm. It will then track your sleep patterns and quality using the microphone on your phone. It's best to do it for at least a week so you get a sense of your baseline sleep quality. Once you've tracked your sleep, you'll have all the data you need to hack your sleep. This will ensure that what you're doing is actually working and allow you to make adjustments along the way based on how you're feeling when you wake up and what the numbers are telling you. To get the best sleep while using an app, you must put your phone in airplane mode. Because the electromagnetic field generated by cell phones interferes with sleep quality, sleeping with an active cell phone near your head will disrupt your sleep whether or not it rings.

The other great thing about Sleep Cycle is that it will act as an alarm clock and wake you at the top of a sleep cycle instead of letting your alarm jerk you awake when you're in a deep sleep. This will leave you feeling more refreshed and awake all day.

As a venture capitalist, I spend most of my time evaluating how technology will change people's lives. I can honestly say that in the last decade, no one has changed my life more than Dave. His Bulletproof Diet has given me more energy and has greatly improved my health and wellbeing. It has been transformational for me and many of the executives I work with in the technology industry. —**Dan Scholnick**

LOW-INTENSITY AMBER BULBS

The light from traditional lightbulbs is known to inhibit the quality of your sleep by shutting off your natural melatonin production. However, your body responds to amber and red light the same way it does to darkness. When you wake up at night to go to the bathroom or nurse your baby, you'll be able to go back to sleep much more quickly if the only light you're exposed to is amber light. You can get amber nightlights online that will help preserve the quality of your sleep.

"ELECTROSLEEP" DEVICE

Cerebral electrical stimulators, or CES devices, have been around since 1949, when the Russians first deployed them on space missions using uniquely Russian logic. The idea was that since it takes a lot of expensive fuel to put an astronaut into space, they could use technology to let astronauts sleep less. That way, they'd pay to send fewer astronauts into space and still get the same amount of work done. This technology is almost 70 years old, but few people have ever heard of it.

I've used CES since 1998, and as I type this my CES device is running a tiny gamma frequency electrical current between my temples. It is a small box about the size of two iPhones that is powered by a 9-volt battery. A small clip attaches to each of my earlobes, and the pulse between my ears tells my brain to get into that specific frequency. Recently I set my CES device to run a carefully shaped, controlled microcurrent across my brain and put it into a deep state of sleep for 45 minutes, the kind of sleep that restores your brain and causes hormones to be released. This forced me to get more deep sleep than I otherwise would have in the only 2½ hours I had to sleep that night. I woke up full of energy and feeling as if I'd slept at least an unhacked 7 or 8 hours. I didn't need any stimulants in the morning, just a single cup of Bulletproof Coffee to make me feel like I could climb a mountain while writing this book. CES is shown to be a safe and effective treatment for insomnia,[21] and it's even been used to treat anxiety and drug addiction. The cost of the device ranges from $300 to $2,000. You can get them online without a prescription, or your insurance provider may cover one if your doctor prescribes it—not that your doctor has likely ever heard of this!

EARTHING MAT

In 2005, I was flying from the West Coast to Cambridge, England, every month because I was an executive for a startup based there. Even with Virgin Airline's awesome seats, the jet lag from flying east was painful. I'd heard about the idea that walking barefoot on grass for a few minutes makes jet lag go away. Being a rational engineer, I laughed at this idea, but I knew that raising body temperature by exercising in the morning is effective for resetting circadian rhythms, so I tried doing yoga in the park by my hotel while barefoot. What an incredible difference! I did not experience the negative effects of jet lag at all. I figured it was the yoga and tried doing yoga indoors on the next trip—the same series at the same time of day—but it did not have the same effect. The biohacker in me was intrigued.

After a few trips, I confirmed for myself that grounding worked for reasons I simply didn't understand. Then a few months later I read about a cable systems engineering entrepreneur turned biohacker who figured out that electrically grounding himself had all kinds of positive effects on circadian rhythm and inflammation. He funded some small studies that showed grounding increases resilience because it speeds recovery, lowers inflammation, and normalizes cortisol.[22]

The theory is that our bodies develop a positive charge that is slowly dispelled when we touch the earth. The earth itself has negatively charged electrons that balance the positive charge we accumulate when we're disconnected, which happens because we are almost always electrically insulated from the surface of the planet. Over time, this positive charge builds up, depletes our energy, and promotes inflammation and disease. Now I usually travel with a small strap that plugs into the grounding outlet in my hotel room because it reliably helps to cure jet lag while I'm sleeping. My mind is clearer when I use it, too. I sleep grounded most of the time at home, too, on a conductive sheet. Sadly, it's not 1,000 thread count, but my awesome wife, Lana (a medical doctor), permits it because she feels the effects on her sleep, too.

SLEEP INDUCTION MAT

Acupressure mats stimulate muscle relaxation by using the power of acupressure points. It is possible to get one formulated as a sleep induction mat, which helps you go to sleep and stay asleep while reducing your muscular aches and pains. Look for one made of nontoxic hemp or organic cotton with big, powerful acupressure points. To use the sleep induction mat, you have to train the Labrador in your head. When you first lie on the spikes, your Labrador brain will be convinced that they're deadly. You'll experience a wave of discomfort as your fight-or-flight response takes over. By taking charge with your human brain and staying on the mat, you'll cause your sympathetic nervous system to relax, and what was incredibly uncomfortable 1 minute ago now feels blissful and relaxing. Simply lying on it for a few minutes will cause a surge of endorphins, a wave of relaxation that you can easily feel, and helps to create very deep sleep that you will often see when tracking your sleep with the Sleep Cycle app.

HEART RATE VARIABILITY MEDITATION

Just breathing or meditating before going to bed can help you sleep better, but you can get even better results when you have technology guiding you to a state where your fight-or-flight response turns off. When your mind is racing, it's hard to go to sleep, and you can waste a lot of time trying to get to sleep if your Labrador brain is running around looking for tigers or searching for food. One of the best ways I've found to turn off that fight-or-flight response is to use heart rate variability training. When you are in a fight-or-flight state, the spacing between your heartbeats gets very even.[23] This is the sign of a stressed animal. When your Labrador brain is calm, the amount of time between each heartbeat changes and becomes more variable. Of course, being out of a fight-or-flight response is correlated with better sleep.

Heart rate variability works both ways—intentionally making your heart rate more variable will calm you down, while naturally calming down will make your heart rate more variable. The Bulletproof Stress Detective app works with a heart rate strap or stick-on sensor to help you know when your stress levels are high throughout the day, and the Heart-Math Inner Balance Sensor uses breathing exercises to teach you what it's like to be out of fight-or-flight and how to quickly turn it off. By looking at a screen during the breathing exercises, you can easily see when you're doing it right. In this way, technology gives you feedback so you can alter your breathing and put yourself in a calm state. I used this technique to learn how to go to sleep in 3 minutes reliably.

The great thing about heart rate variability training is that you can do it almost anywhere at any time, and it gives you objective data on how much you've improved. If you're having trouble sleeping, try a few minutes of heart rate variability training before bed, using either Stress Detective or HeartMath. Even 5 minutes is sometimes enough to put the most tweaked-out executives to sleep. I use these simple techniques with my clients to improve performance and sleep.

WHAT TO AVOID

It's just as important to avoid doing the wrong things before going to bed as it is to do the right things. Here are the most important things to avoid at night in order to get the best possible quality sleep.

BRIGHT LIGHTS

For at least a half hour before going to bed, try to avoid bright lights. Dim your office lights if you absolutely must be working this close to bedtime, and kill the unhealthy flourescent ones. You can also install free software called f.lux on your PC or Mac to automatically dim the screen at night; I've used this software with great results for nearly a decade. Don't stare at your TV, cell phone, or tablet until you've dimmed it all the way, either. Even 5 minutes of white light from a screen shuts off your melatonin production for hours and can wreck the quality of your sleep, so it's best to avoid screens in the evening entirely.

VIOLENCE

Watching graphic violence on TV might make it harder for you to fall and stay asleep. Watching violence tends to get the Labrador in your brain looking for threats, and when you try to go to sleep it's harder to get out of fight-or-flight mode. If you ignore this advice and watch it anyway, try using the HeartMath Inner Balance Sensor for a few minutes to reverse the effects and get out of fight-or-flight so you can fall asleep.

EXERCISE

You should not exercise for at least 2 hours before going to bed, unless you count restorative yoga and breathing exercises as exercise. Sleep and exercise are intimately connected, as I'll discuss more in the next chapter. Exercise is highly energizing and raises your cortisol levels, which interferes with sleep. Don't hack your sleep after exercising!

CAFFEINE

Drinking Bulletproof Coffee puts your mind in an amazing place where you become more productive and perform better. However, you need to let your mind rest after its high-output performances. In general, don't drink coffee after 2:00 p.m. or at least 8 hours before bedtime, whichever comes first. This will make sure you get all of the cognitive benefits of caffeine without sacrificing your sleep. Some people need more than 8 hours of caffeine avoidance for maximum performance sleep. Keep track of your caffeine intake and sleep patterns to see how it affects you.

SECOND WIND

There is a window from 10:45 and 11:00 p.m. or so when you naturally get tired. This moves a little bit based on the season. If you don't go to sleep then and choose to stay awake, you'll get a cortisol-driven "second wind" that can keep you awake until 2:00 a.m. You'll also get better sleep when you go to bed before 11:00 p.m. and wake up feeling more rested than if you'd gotten the same amount of sleep starting later. I'll be the first to admit that I'm almost never in bed before 11:00 p.m., but it's good to know about this second wind so you can choose to either avoid it or take advantage of it. When working to support my adrenal glands, I slept from 10:00 p.m. to 5:00 a.m. for 18 months straight. But I've always done my best research, coding, and writing after 11:00 p.m., so I choose to take advantage of the second wind and use it to get more done on fewer hours of highly efficient sleep.

STRESS

Stress can be a good thing when it is motivational or causes positive change. Life is boring without useful stress such as reaching for a goal or making a constructive life change, but nonbeneficial stress is terribly wasteful. It not only decreases immune function, shortens your life span, and impairs sexual performance, but also destroys your sleep. Perhaps the most common reason people report not being able to sleep is that they don't know how to clear their minds and stop worrying. Deep-breathing exercises like Art of Living, pranayama yoga, and meditation can do wonders for helping your brain shut down, recuperate, and prepare for another day of Bulletproof high performance.

If you want to start measuring your own stress, download the Bulletproof Stress Detective app here:

 http://bulletproofexec.com/
stress-detective-ios

 http://bulletproofexec.com/
stress-detective-android

When you get right down to it, food is the most important variable that makes an impact on energy levels and weight loss and can keep the Labrador in your head happy. The second most important variable, which is even more important than exercise, is the quality of your sleep. You don't need to use all of the tools outlined in this chapter, but changing what you eat before you sleep and becoming conscious of the quality of your sleep can give you an edge in how well your diet works for you.

CHAPTER

6

WORK OUT LESS AND GET MORE MUSCLE

Like most people, I used to believe that exercising a *lot* was the best way to get the body I wanted. I forced myself to work out 6 days a week for 90 minutes at a time, and then told myself I was a great human being for doing that. But despite my self-assurances and the certainty that I was doing the right thing, I didn't drop the fat I wanted to lose. I did get stronger and faster, but not thinner. Imagine my horror (and biohacking delight!) when I discovered years later that the exercise I'd been doing was wasteful because I was doing too much, doing it too frequently, and doing it for too long.

If your goal is to be in a state of high performance where you feel good and have lots of free energy, spending your time on excessive non-productive exercise just uses up your willpower and burdens your body with extra stress, but it doesn't help you live a longer or healthier life. To top it off, exercise is not even the biggest factor in determining what your body looks like. Since 80 to 90 percent of what your body looks like depends on what you eat, most people can get a lean, strong body with virtually no exercise at all. It only takes a few simple hacks.

Don't get me wrong—doing the right exercise is extremely beneficial. It grows your brain capacity by releasing a protein that interacts with hormones called BDNF (brain-derived neurotrophic factor), helps increase insulin sensitivity, reduces cardiac risk, and burns off stress.[1] Unfortunately, most people do it wrong, for too long, and don't allow their muscles to recover.

As you've already read, your body composition is not primarily determined by the amount of calories you eat. In fact, hormones (and gut bacteria) determine the shape of your body. It therefore makes sense to view exercise as another tool in your arsenal that lets you control your hormones, just like sleep or food. We've already learned that when you use biohacking, you can get far more benefits in less time. Why should exercise be any different?

Overtraining and under-recovering is a common problem among my type-A business executive clients. The same drive that makes someone want

As an endurance athlete living above the Arctic Circle, I am always at battle with extreme conditions. Long-distance dog racing requires mushers to be fully alert for days on end with little to no sleep. They must not only care for themselves but [also] up to 16 canine companions. The low temperatures and low sunlight demand much energy from the racers. In other words—we must be Bulletproof! I am also an Ironman triathlete trying to qualify for the world championships. There is not much sitting still, but when I do sit I am at the computer consulting as an energy engineer, and my brain must work despite the fatigue. The Bulletproof products have seen me through a trying winter. Every morning I wake up with my Bulletproof Coffee with grass-fed butter and Brain Octane oil. My favorite lunch consists of a coconut milk smoothie with [Upgraded] whey protein and cacao butter. As I have transferred to a ketogenic diet following the Bulletproof Diet principles, I have relied heavily on Brain Octane Oil for fueling. During workouts, I mix a tablespoon of Brain Octane Oil with UCAN SuperStarch, and finally eliminated my previously challenging gut issues. **—Katherine Keith** to run a company can also make them want to complete an Ironman triathlon. But all that exercise on top of a stressful job will drive up your cortisol levels. This causes weight gain, muscle loss, a decline in testosterone, and burnout. That's not only what the research shows, but also exactly what happened to me. At the age of 30, I had the testosterone level of a 50-year-old man, the estrogen level of a middle-aged woman, and stress hormone levels nearly 10 times higher than the level that triggers burnout.

Being Bulletproof means using the most efficient techniques that get the job done with minimal effort and in the smallest amount of time.

When done moderately and correctly, exercise improves bone density, mood, and blood lipids, and increases insulin sensitivity and lean muscle. It can also decrease inflammation and help you sleep better, as long as it's done more than 2 hours before you go to bed. It is possible to stay lean and muscular while doing excessive exercise on a starvation diet or while doing no exercise on the Bulletproof Diet, but the best long-term and short-term results come from following the diet while doing just enough exercise to reach your goals. From a Bulletproof perspective, that means using the most efficient techniques that get the job done with minimal effort and in the smallest amount of time.

If you're not satisfied with simply being lean and muscular and want to look like a ripped god or goddess, it's going to take a little more exercise and a lot more recovery. I'll be perfectly honest—I want to live a very long time with a brain that never quits and a body that relentlessly fights aging. And I want to look good while doing it, but not necessarily as good as a chiseled movie star. That's because my other goal is to spend my days doing things I love with people I care about. For example, I consciously chose to put my energy into writing this book so more people can benefit from the Bullet-proof Diet instead of spending my time recovering from a more intense exercise regimen. You can use these techniques to build whatever type of body you like. And by the way, the biohacking advice in this book actually does work for chiseled movie stars, Hollywood celebrities, world champion athletes, MMA fighters, and CrossFit and Ironman athletes.

> I am a high-performing Ironman triathlete. I have used the Bulletproof nutritional protocols as well as Dave's supplements to produce superior results. I recently finished in the top 5 percent of all finishers at Ironman Texas with Dave's help. As part of my training, his recommendations allowed me to shift from a carb burner to a fat burner. **—Adam Brennen, wealth strategist**

First, let's define what I mean by "exercise." To quote Doug McGuff, MD, a friend, physician, exercise physiologist, gifted biohacker, and author of *Body by Science,* "Exercise is a specific activity that stimulates a positive physiological adaptation that serves to enhance fitness and health. It does not undermine the latter in the process of enhancing the former." This means that in order for you to use exercise as a tool to sculpt your body and build a more resilient life, it must be brief, intense, infrequent, safe, and purposeful.

Anything that does not meet these criteria is not exercise. Marathons, Ironmans, ultra-endurance events, long jogging routes, and any form of excessive heavy lifting are not quite exercise based on these criteria for the simple fact that they do not optimize health while creating fitness. They are immensely challenging and require admirable physical and mental strength, but they are not exercise the way we're defining it unless they increase your health and fitness. No matter how fit and ripped you are or how good your backside looks in yoga pants, you won't achieve Bulletproof resilience and power unless you're healthy.

As we've seen from the heart scarring and temporary damage that come from running marathons,[2] being fit or being able to compete in a specific sport does not mean that you are healthy. A small 2010 study designed to figure out why people occasionally drop dead of heart attacks during marathons reveals evidence that extreme chronic cardio actually strains the heart and causes damage to the heart muscle,[3] but exercise should reduce your cardiovascular risk if it's improving your health. The good news is that by understanding that your chosen sport may be potentially harmful to your body, especially if you are overtrained or undertrained, you can often use biohacking techniques to minimize the harm and maximize your recovery.

At the opposite end of the spectrum, choosing the stairs over the elevator or taking a lunchtime walk or leisurely bike ride isn't really exercise either because it isn't intense and doesn't cause a direct physiological adaptation. This is merely moving around. You won't get the hormonal effects of real exercise from these activities, but you'll still benefit from them. Moving decreases your risk of metabolic syndrome,[4] breast cancer,[5] cardiovascular disease,[6] and vascular dementia.[7] It also decreases overall systemic inflammation,[8] which saps your performance and contributes to almost all known diseases. Moderate physical activity also likely decreases the number of upper respiratory tract infections you get[9] and improves mood in people who are depressed.[10] In healthy people, easy movement can improve mood for up to 2 hours afterward.[11] It also improves mitochondrial function,[12] which, as you've read, helps your brain perform better. So go for a walk, but don't fool yourself into thinking you exercised when all you did was walk!

Weight training is the most Bulletproof form of exercise because it meets all of the requirements for proper exercise, increases your lean muscle mass, boosts your insulin sensitivity and metabolic rate for days, and increases your testosterone and growth hormone levels (including healthy amounts for women). Not only is having more muscle good for your health because it makes you more resilient to fatigue, diseases, pathogens, and toxins, but it will also allow you to perform with more

My boyfriend and I competed this past weekend at a bodybuilding competition and used your XCT Oil, Brain Octane Oil, and Bulletproof Coffee practically every day during our 14-week prep. We felt amazing and were able to maintain and even build muscle while cutting our body fat. We even kept the Brain Octane backstage for fuel during the show. We feel amazing, and I took home second place at the most competitive amateur bodybuilding competition in history against over 748 athletes!
—Alexis

confidence and pride on a daily basis. Within limits, muscle mass generates health in both men and women.

Some people shy away from weight training, but everyone from stay-at-home moms to elite athletes and entrepreneurs can benefit from being stronger. Women should not worry that weight lifting will cause them to "bulk up"! Weight training is the recommended form of exercise for anyone who wants to cut fat and gain muscle. Don't be fooled into believing that traditional cardio is necessary for improving cardiovascular function. In many cases, long workouts of cardio practiced for the wrong reasons (to "burn" calories) are detrimental to your health because they stress the heart and body but don't cause the beneficial change exercise should.

It is impossible to isolate one aspect of fitness (such as your cardiovascular system, muscular system, aerobic system, etc.), nor would you want to, but many people believe they must isolate their cardiovascular system by doing "cardio" workouts. Typical cardio workouts like running or cycling do count as exercise in that they increase health, but most aren't efficient enough. Fortunately, there is a way to use biohacking to get a strong heart and lungs, the main benefits of cardio workouts, in minimal amounts of time. It is called high-intensity interval training. To do this, you only need a place where you can run a few hundred meters. Simply run as fast as you can, like a tiger is chasing your inner Labrador. Run for 30 seconds, rest for 90 seconds, and then do it again. Repeat this until 15 minutes have passed. If you're like most people who don't do this often, you won't last 15 minutes on your first shot. That's okay. Work up to it.

The benefits? You'll produce more human growth hormone (HGH), the performance-enhancing antiaging hormone your body makes to keep you young. One study found that doing an intense workout like this for at least 10 minutes caused the greatest secretion of HGH.[13] Another study found that the more intense the exercise, the more intense the HGH release.[14] So go ahead, run like something's chasing you. Your heart and lungs will benefit and could help you live longer. Best of all, you can do this once a week for 15 minutes and get more cardio benefits that you

DOES IT MATTER WHEN I EXERCISE?

It took some experimenting to find out what time of day exercising gave me the best results and what to eat before and after working out. When I worked out for 1½ hours a day 6 days a week, I often did so at 9:00 or 10:00 at night because that's when I had time. This didn't give me the results I was looking for. I also tried working out in the morning, which some people like because it fits into their work-day. The problem with this is that your cortisol naturally spikes in the morning, so exercising (which also raises cortisol) at this time may cause a higher spike in cortisol than is recommended by health professionals.

I finally found my answer when I learned about mTOR (mammalian target of rapamycin) and the three things that cause it to be suppressed and then bounce back to build muscle: coffee, fasting, and exercise. I realized the way to get the best results was to stack my mTOR suppression by using every possible way to tamp it down it so I'd get the biggest surge and most muscle gain afterward. This is why I get the best results from exercising right near the end of my Bulletproof Intermittent Fast. I eat dinner, go to sleep, and enjoy Bulletproof Coffee for breakfast. Several hours later, at around 1:00 or 2:00 p.m., I exercise, and then I eat a high-vegetable, high-protein, and high-fat meal. That night I have extra carbs with dinner. A 2010 Belgian study demonstrated for the first time that exercising on an empty stomach (in a fasted state) while on a high-fat diet with plenty of calories—like the Bulletproof Diet—provides the most muscle growth, improves whole body glucose tolerance, and improves insulin sensitivity.[15]

I also recommend supplementing with a high-quality protein source like grass-fed hydrolyzed collagen protein or cold processed whey concentrate protein within 15 minutes of finishing a workout to prevent a muscle-robbing cortisol spike that can last for up to 48 hours. The collagen is especially good for you because it makes your skin and ligaments more flexible, too.

would from a daily 1-hour jog! You really can trade intensity for time with exercise, whether it's sprinting or lifting. Do this once a week and at least 3 days before or after lifting weights.

When it comes to lifting weights, it's best to work out one to three times per week (in addition to the interval training). You should only train three times a week if you have extra time for sleep and recovery and are not jet-lagged. If you find your training stalling on this program, decrease the frequency instead of forcing yourself to try harder. Remember, there is a point of diminishing returns with exercise. More exercise will not always lead to more benefits, and overtraining is harmful.

Each workout should not last longer than 20 minutes. Often, 10 to 15 minutes is enough, but your workout should be extremely high intensity, with each movement done to the point of muscle failure. This is the when the weight won't move anymore no matter how hard you tell your Labrador brain to move it. Unless you're working with a trainer or experienced with free weights, it's best to start with using machines, as pushing yourself to muscle fatigue with free weights increases your risk of injury. The weight should be heavy enough that you will reach muscle failure in $1\frac{1}{2}$ to 2 minutes. A good rule is to use about 80 percent of the heaviest amount of weight you're capable of lifting one time. The next movement should be performed as soon as possible after the completion of the previous one. The time between movements should not exceed 2 minutes, and less is better.

The five compound movements that are most beneficial are:

Seated row
Chest press
Pulldown
Overhead press
Leg press

There's some debate among fitness experts about how much you should warm up. Some stretching is fine, but you don't have to go for a jog or do jumping jacks to warm up. You can do these movements in whatever

PLAN TO EXERCISE

For more details about exercise, I highly recommend the following books:

Enter the Kettlebell! Strength Secret of the Soviet Supermen, by Pavel Tsatsouline (St. Paul, MN: Dragon Door, 2006)

Pavel Tsatsouline is the godfather of kettlebell training, and if you want an intense workout, there's no better way than with kettlebells. I've had kettlebells in my office for years, and I still use them occasionally when I have time. This is a great workout and a great guide for people who are looking to achieve the next level of fitness.

Starting Strength: Basic Barbell Training (3rd ed.), by Mark Rippetoe (Wichita Falls, TX: Aasgaard, 2013)

Body by Science, by Doug McGuff and John Little (New York: McGraw-Hill, 2009)

This book is all about how to get the most benefit in the least amount of time. It is not for hard-core bodybuilders. It's for people who want to look and feel good, live regular lives, and be Bulletproof.

Becoming a Supple Leopard: The Ultimate Guide to Resolving Pain, Preventing Injury, and Optimizing Athletic Performance, by Kelly Starrett and Glen Cordoza (Las Vegas: Victory Belt, 2013)

This book focuses on the movement side of exercise and is a must-read. Plus, author Kelly Starrett is the person who first came up with the term "disaster pants."

The Four-Hour Body, by Timothy Ferriss (New York: Crown, 2010)

This book has amazing advice about using minimal amounts of exercise for very rapid gains. It also does a great job of teaching you how to track your body fat and muscle to make sure your exercise plan is working for you.

order you prefer. Perform each one for 1½ to 2 minutes (until you couldn't do another one to save your life). If you've never tried these exercises before, that's okay. Go to a local gym and hire a trainer for one session to show you how to do them properly. They are simple exercises. Another option is to find a local CrossFit gym (called a box), where a trainer will teach you the equivalents of these movements using free weights. Just explain that you are new to this and want a very short workout, and you'll do fine. Expect to be very sore after these workouts, and start with just once a week so you have time to recover and build muscle before starting over.

Keep in mind that proper recovery is extremely important. Whether you perform the weight-lifting exercise or the high-intensity interval training sprints, make sure you wait at the very least for 2 days and up to 10 days before your next workout. Between 4 and 7 days is the sweet spot. Eating some extra Bulletproof carbs on the evening of your workout day will help you recover faster. Bodybuilders have been eating carbs after workouts for decades. Carbs do increase insulin, but insulin's job is to carry protein and fat into your muscles. When you stimulate your muscles through exercise, you do want to have some insulin to feed them, but not too much. This is another example of how you can carefully time your carbs to get the best results.

Remember, your diet is more important than exercise in determining the shape of your body and how you feel. These exercises are simply a way for you to become stronger and more powerful. For nonathletes, I recommend weight lifting once during week 1, sprinting once during week 2, and then repeating. That comes to only four workouts a month. The night after you exercise, you need to sleep much more than someone who is sedentary because muscle tissue is repaired during deep sleep. A 20-minute workout can increase your sleep needs by more than 3 hours a night. If you're exercising more than two times per week, let your body sleep as much as it needs. *Never* work out more than once a week if you're restricting your sleep, and don't do heavy workouts when you're jet-lagged. Your job is to be a recovery machine, not an exercise machine. Remember, the recovery is when your body builds muscle!

7

WEAK MULTIVITAMINS AND THE BULLETPROOF GUIDE TO SUPPLEMENTS

A s the standard American diet has shifted away from foods that are high in nutrients like healthy animal protein and vegetables and we've come to rely more on nutritionally void grains, processed foods, and low-fat dairy from poorly fed animals, micronutrient deficiency has become a widespread epidemic. People today are consuming fewer nutrients than ever.[1] To paraphrase journalist, author, and food activist Michael Pollan, the world is becoming overfed and undernourished. Forty-eight percent of the US population is deficient in magnesium,[2] 40 percent are deficient in vitamin B_{12},[3] and 10 percent are deficient in folate.[4]

This is no small matter, as micronutrient deficiencies chip away at your performance long before they cause disease. They cause DNA damage, making you age faster and die sooner.[5] In fact, almost every common disease has been linked to micronutrient deficiencies. When you are deficient in nutrients, your cells don't perform very well. Plus, your Labrador brain thinks it's starving and begs you to eat all sorts of weird things. As a result, micronutrient deficiencies cause fatigue and poor sleep and degrade your mental performance. No matter how much food you consume, it's impossible to live up to your full potential as a human being without the right nutrients. If your "human hardware" is not working at the cellular level, you have little chance of making your "software" do its best. Your Labrador brain won't rest when you are lacking key nutrients, but the cause is hard to determine when it's a hidden vitamin deficiency.

It's no wonder why so many people want to fix this situation with a single pill, but these "only one pill per day" mash-up multivitamins are usually some of the worst forms of supplements on the market. Nearly every antiaging physician I've worked with or interviewed uses vitamins and supplements as primary tools to get results with patients, but none of them recommends the commonly available multivitamins. Most are ineffective, and some are poor formulations that actually cause more harm than good by providing an imbalance of nutrients. They have too much of some (such as vitamin A or B_6) and not enough of others (like magnesium). The result is that you overdose and underdose at the same time.

It's also common practice among most multivitamin manufacturers to include very small amounts of more expensive nutrients. This way they can still be listed on the label. Average consumers often don't notice or can't tell that their pill contains only trace amounts of some nutrients. Their main concern is that they only have to take one pill, but there is no way to fit the correct dosage of "a complete spectrum" of nutrients into one single pill. The Recommended Dietary Allowance (RDA) of magnesium alone, for instance, is larger than will fit in the capsule size of most common multivitamins.

Another issue with multivitamins is that the nutrients they contain are often low quality. Nutrients come in different forms that behave quite differently inside your body. Folate is an essential B vitamin, but consuming high doses of folic acid—the synthetic form of folate—that is found in most multivitamins and fortified foods actually increases your risk of cancer,[6] and some of the population has a common genetic mutation that makes it hard for their bodies to use that form of folic acid. It is common to use yeast-based ingredients as well, which are cheaper but tend to worsen yeast infection problems in people who take them. This may be why many studies show no benefit to taking multivitamins, and much of the research actually reveals an increased risk of mortality associated with them.[7]

Many multivitamins are also made with fillers and additives that make the pills easy to produce but difficult for the body to absorb. Manufacturers also often use shellac (a different kind than the one you find in hardware stores) or other substances to seal off the vitamins from air and moisture before you take them, but this also makes them harder for the pill to disintegrate in the body. This means that even if the correct amount of a nutrient is listed on the label, very little of it may actually reach your cells.[8]

It's always better to get a high-quality version of a nutrient that your body can readily absorb than it is to make up for what's lacking in your diet by taking a pill. The nutrients in food work together in a process known as food synergy. For example, the nutrients digested from a piece of meat are more bioavailable than they are when you consume the same nutrients from a pill, because your body knows how to break down the nutrients in food better than the ones found in vitamins. Studies have shown that eating grass-fed meat boosts plasma omega-3 levels far more than can be explained by the amount of omega-3s in the meat.[9] Meanwhile, antioxidants consumed from foods are usually beneficial, but taking megadoses of some synthetic antioxidants—like isolated synthetic vitamin E fractions—increases your risk of death.[10] In short, this means that food is more powerful than the sum of its parts. Maybe someday we will understand how nutrients interact when they're combined, but right now most studies look at the effects of isolated nutrients. The best thing you can do to live a long time is to eat the highest-quality food.

When it comes to supplements, you definitely get what you pay for. You can delude yourself and buy the generic multivitamins at the big-box stores that are full of fillers and insignificant amounts of important, more expensive nutrients, or spend a little extra and buy targeted supplements that will actually boost your performance. This doesn't mean that you should use supplements to replace a healthy diet, even when they're the highest-quality, most-targeted supplements. Your first goal should be to get as many vitamins and nutrients as possible from your food on the Bulletproof Diet and then to push your performance over the edge with properly selected, timed, and measured supplements. When you get this right, your body and brain will thrive, allowing you to perform at levels you never knew you were capable of.

One of the most common criticisms of this type of targeted supplementation is that the body may not absorb them, but taking these supplements with foods that contain fats helps a lot, because many nutrients need fat to help your body absorb them properly. In fact, adding fat to your vegetables (or coffee) helps you absorb their vitamins, too! When you do that, you don't need to be afraid of wasting money on supplements you can't absorb. Worst-case scenario, you end up with expensive pee. In fact, one of my goals as a biohacker is to have expensive pee. I want my body to have more than enough of all the vitamins and minerals it needs (but not in excessive amounts). Think about it this way—expensive pee is a lot cheaper than cardiac surgery.

RECOMMENDED SUPPLEMENTS

After a decade of running the nonprofit Silicon Valley Health Institute antiaging group, working on *Bulletproof Radio* with countless physicians who use supplements with their patients, and trying just about every supplement on earth, I believe that these are the 10 most important basic supplements that most people should be taking to enhance their diets for optimum performance. I take a lot more, but this list is the "low-hanging vegetable" (who wants sugary fruit, anyway?) list of supplements that have amazing cost-benefit ratio.

For each nutrient below I've provided a dosage recommendation, the correct form it should be taken in, and the time of day it should be taken. I do recommend certain high-quality brands above others, but this list often changes as various companies alter their practices. For the most up-to-date recommendations, please visit bulletproofexec.com/top10. Please note that I have no affiliation with these companies. I am pleased to offer some powerful and unusual Bulletproof supplements on my Web site, but they aren't the commonly available ones on this list. You do not need to buy the Bulletproof brand or share your hard-earned dollars with me in order to benefit from these supplements.

Please be aware that different individuals require varying amounts of each supplement. For example, athletes need to supplement more than average people, as do people who are significantly overweight. The dosages I've set out are good starting points for most people, but it's always best to check with your doctor and get your blood tested for exact nutrient levels so that you can customize your supplement plan and make sure you are getting the right dose. You may notice that these recommended dosages are generally higher than the government's RDAs. After 10 years of working with health professionals who use vitamins to make people healthier and seeing profound results myself, it has become painfully obvious to me that many of the RDAs were determined simply to prevent disease or death due to vitamin deficiency. For example, the amount of vitamin C you need to avoid scurvy is much less than the amount you

My son had tremendous success with his weight loss and health on the Bulletproof Diet. I tagged along! I'm wheat-free for a year and taking every supplement on the list! No more asthma or blood pressure meds!
—Charlotte

need to thrive. Avoiding death is great and all, but living up to your full potential is even better. That's what these recommended dosages should help you achieve.

VITAMIN D

Vitamin D isn't just the most important supplement, it's probably the most important biohack from the world of antiaging and human performance. You've already learned how important adequate levels of vitamin D are when it comes to your sleep, but vitamin D also acts on more than 1,000 different genes and serves as a substrate for hormones like testosterone, human growth hormone, and estrogen. It moderates immune function and inflammation and assists in calcium metabolism and bone formation. I found that I got sick far less often when I started taking vitamin D. It's no coincidence that this is one of the few vitamins humans can make on their own, just from sunlight and cholesterol. Without it, we'd be dead. While it is possible to get adequate vitamin D from sun exposure, if you don't live near the equator and aren't a nudist, chances are you aren't getting enough.

> **Dose:** 1,000 IU for every 25 pounds of body weight
> **Form:** D_3
> **Time to Take:** Morning

Note: People with darker skin don't convert sunlight into vitamin D as quickly as those with lighter skin. If you're dark-skinned, a safe bet is 1,500 IU for every 25 pounds of body weight, but you should always test your blood levels because individual responses to dosage vary. If you are pregnant or planning to become pregnant, having adequate vitamin D is critical to your baby's long-term health.

MAGNESIUM

Magnesium is almost as important as vitamin D and almost as underappreciated. Magnesium is used in more than 300 enzymatic processes, so low magnesium means low cellular energy. It's also vital for proper transcription of DNA and RNA. Magnesium deficiency is a serious problem. Symptoms include heart arrhythmias such as tachycardia (when the heart beats abnormally fast), headaches, muscle cramps, nausea, metabolic syndrome, migraines, and pretty much everything else you don't want. It's also associated with cardiovascular disease, diabetes, asthma, anxiety disorders, and PMS. To put it simply, magnesium makes the body more resilient to stress. For someone who wants to be able to withstand more stress, magnesium is an obvious supplement to take.

Amazingly, based on the RDA, almost all Americans are deficient in magnesium, although even that amount is thought to be too low.[11] Magnesium should be present in adequate amounts in vegetables, which absorb it from the soil, but soil depletion and poor farming practices have made it almost impossible to get enough magnesium from your diet alone. Without a doubt, everyone should supplement with magnesium.

Dose: 600 to 800 mg per day

Form: Citrate, malate, aspartate, glycinate, threonate, or orotate

Time to Take: Bedtime

VITAMIN K_2

Unless you grew up eating only grass-fed meat and raw milk, you're probably deficient in vitamin K_2. People think they can get vitamin K from eating vegetables, but there are two types of vitamin K—K_1 and K_2. It's easiest to think of vitamin K_1 and vitamin K_2 as two entirely different vitamins. Vitamin K_1 is found in leafy vegetables like kale, while vitamin K_2 is found in grass-fed animal products. Ruminant animals like cows and sheep convert K_1 into K_2 in their stomachs, but humans don't convert vitamin K_1 into K_2 very efficiently. This is yet another reason that you should eat grass-fed animals—cows need grass in their diet to produce K_2 in their milk.

K_2 is a fat-soluble vitamin that helps with calcium metabolism. When calcium isn't properly metabolized, excess calcium is deposited in arteries, leading to calcification and decreased vascular function. This is why vitamin K_2 helps to prevent atherosclerosis and heart attacks while strengthening bones. Since vitamin D helps metabolize calcium, vitamins D and K_2 work together synergistically. You won't benefit as much from vitamin D if you don't have enough K_2.

There are two subsets of vitamin K_2: MK-4 and MK-7. MK-4 is the kind shown to produce the most benefit, but MK-7 is still important. MK-4 comes from animal sources, which is best. MK-7 comes from intestinal bacterial fermentation, which isn't as effective. You should consume a total of 2,000 micrograms (mcg) per day of K_2, at least 100 mcg of which should be in the MK-7 form. Supplements with MK-4 in them often come from an extract of tobacco, so it's especially important to take supplements with MK-7. An even better way to get it is to eat a lot of butter!

Dose: 2,000 mcg per day (100 mcg as MK-7)

Form: MK-4, MK-7

Time to Take: For this vitamin it doesn't really matter, but since it's best to take K_2 with vitamin D because they work together synergistically, you should take it in the morning.

VITAMIN C

This is one of the safest, most effective supplements you can take. Vitamin C is needed for the formation of collagen and connective tissue as well as for manufacturing glutathione, the most powerful antioxidant in the body. Vitamin C can enhance immune function and help prevent free radical damage.

It's hard to get enough vitamin C from food. Some fruits and vegetables are naturally high in vitamin C, like broccoli, cauliflower, and of course oranges. But cooking and storage methods can deplete it in many foods. This is why about 20 percent of the population is vitamin C deficient.[12]

While studies have shown that you can take up to 120 grams of vitamin C a day with no side effects other than loose stool,[13] your body can often tolerate a lot more when it's sick or under stress. The more sick or stressed you are, the more C you can tolerate without getting to a "disaster pants" level of stool softness. I've done some ridiculous biohacks with vitamin C. When I realized how badly antibiotics had messed up my gut, I was determined to never take them again. Anytime I got sick after that, I turned to extremely high doses of vitamin C to cure me. One time I got a massive sinus infection, probably the worst one of my life. I took 100 grams of vitamin C orally, which is an extremely high dose, and then went to a doctor who agreed to administer an additional 150 grams via IV. Even this high dose didn't give me loose stools, which means my body was using all of it to fight the infection. If your body is stressed, it will drink vitamin C like water, so take extra if you're having a rough day, traveling, or feeling under the weather.

Dose: 1 to 2 g per day (more if you are suffering from chronic infections or healing after an injury)

Form: Ascorbic acid crystals or time-release capsules

Time to Take: Morning and evening, but not after a workout since isolated antioxidants can negate the insulin sensitivity gained from exercise

The only time I used to take vitamins C and D was when I started to feel sick and would "megadose" on them for a few days. Since starting the Bulletproof Diet, I supplement with C and D daily, along with K_2 and iodine and then magnesium at night. I cannot remember the last time I was sick, and I believe it is thanks to healthier eating and supplementing. Also, I have better and deeper sleep when I take magnesium before bed. **—Greg**

IODINE

Iodine is crucial for proper thyroid function and metabolism, so this is an important supplement to take when you're trying to lose weight. It also enhances immune function and prevents brain damage. Though you can get iodine from seafood and iodized salt, it is difficult to get an optimal level from food, and iodine deficiency is widespread.

Dose: 1 mg per day
Form: Kelp powder or potassium iodide capsules
Time to Take: Doesn't matter

EPA/DHA (KRILL OIL)

It's important to know that not all fish oil is created equal. Small doses of high-quality fish oil can reduce inflammation, improve brain function, and even enhance muscle growth, but poor quality or high doses can cause more problems than they help to solve. Most of the brands you are likely to see at your local grocery store are contaminated, oxidized, and low potency. If you can't find a good fish oil, you're much better off avoiding it altogether.

This is why I recommend krill oil over fish oil. Krill is more stable and is phosphorylated, meaning it's easier for your brain to use. Your body has to naturally phosphatize regular fish oil, so krill saves your body this step. It also comes with astaxanthin, a potent antioxidant. There are real benefits to taking EPA and DHA, which are both omega-3 fatty acids. EPA reduces inflammation, while DHA makes cell membranes, primarily in the brain. They are both in fish and krill oil. The benefits of DHA and EPA are strongest if your diet is deficient in omega-3s or too high in omega-6s. Ideally, your omega-6–to–omega-3 ratio is no more than 4:1. If you're following the Bulletproof Diet, this won't be a problem. Humans only need 350 mg of DHA and EPA a day for optimal brain function. If you're eating grass-fed meat and wild-caught fish, this goal is easily obtainable.

Otherwise, you should supplement with at least 1,000 mg of krill oil per day. If you are using doses above what is recommended here, you should take a small amount of gamma-linolenic acid (GLA) because DHA can lessen the body's natural production of it, but you need it to make some anti-inflammatory compounds.

Dose: 350 to 1,000 mg per day
Form: Krill oil
Time to Take: With meals

VITAMIN A

This is an essential supplement if you aren't eating organ meats like beef liver, kidney, and heart (though you really should be consuming these Bulletproof foods). Vitamin A is an important cofactor for numerous metabolic reactions and bodily functions, but a quarter of Americans consume less than half the RDA of vitamin A, which is already too low.[14] Many people forget that you can't get vitamin A from plants. Plants don't contain vitamin A; they have beta-carotene, which is poorly converted into vitamin A. This is why some populations develop vitamin A deficiency while at the same time consuming far more beta-carotene than they require. Sorry, vegetarians and vegans—in this case, carrots don't count!

Dose: 10,000 to 15,000 IU per day

Form: Retinol (a good source of vitamin A is cod liver oil—which also contains vitamin D—but not enough to provide all you need)

Time to Take: With meals

SELENIUM

Selenium is a heavy metal that has numerous beneficial effects. It boosts immune function, helps prevent cancer and neurodegenerative diseases, and protects against thyroid dysfunction. While it is possible to get enough selenium from wild-caught fish and animal products, most people don't. It's important to be careful with this one and get your blood levels tested, as too much selenium can cause negative health consequences such as kidney, heart, and nervous system problems.

> **Dose:** 200 mcg per day
> **Form:** Se-methylselenocysteine or selenomethionine
> **Time to Take:** Doesn't matter

COPPER

Copper is needed for proper vascular and heart function, but most of the US population is woefully deficient, consuming only an average of 1 mg per day.[15] This is extremely worrying since getting less than 1 mg of copper per day can cause heart attacks. Copper intake has fallen over the last century due to modern farming techniques and dietary practices. Because we have depleted our soil through industrial agriculture, modern fruits, vegetables, and conventional meats are low in copper, containing much less than they used to.

Luckily, beef and lamb liver both have massive amounts of copper. You can meet your copper needs by eating at least 4 ounces of beef liver per week. Other good sources of copper include cocoa (look for low-toxin dark chocolate), cashews, and lobster. I dislike the taste of liver, so I take grass-fed desiccated liver capsules daily.

> **Dose:** 1 mg per day
> **Form:** Capsule
> **Time to Take:** Doesn't matter

VITAMIN B$_{12}$ AND FOLATE

Most people are deficient in Vitamin B$_{12}$, which is found in many animal products and can protect against dementia, increase immune function, maintain nerves, and regenerate cells. One of the inflammatory markers that should go down on the Bulletproof Diet is homocysteine, but if you're low in B_{12} and folate, its level is more likely to remain high. One of the most crucial areas for B_{12} is the brain. Vitamin B_{12} is linked to folate, which is found in plants. They are both required for mental function, and a deficiency in one produces a deficiency in the other because both folate and B_{12} are required for a reaction called transmethylation, which is required to make neurotransmitters like serotonin. If you're low in either B_{12} or folate, your body will use up the other one to attempt to complete this reaction. This is why taking extra folate will not correct a B_{12} deficiency in the brain, and treating a vitamin B_{12} deficiency with folate can result in permanent brain damage. (Do you hear that, vegans?) Likewise, high amounts of folate without adequate B_{12} consumption can cause neurological problems. This is why I take them together.

It is critically important that you choose the forms recommended below, because many people have a common genetic mutation that does not allow them to process folic acid, which is added to foods labeled as "fortified," such as some grains.[16] People with this genetic makeup can't convert folic acid to folate, and so folic acid builds up in their bloodstream and interrupts cellular metabolism. It will be a good day for everyone when government standards require folate instead of folic acid to be added to our foods. In the meantime, everyone should take the types listed below unless they know they have the genes needed to process folic acid.

Dose: 5 mg methylcobalamin or hydroxycobalamin and 800 mcg folate (5-MTHF or folinic acid, NOT folic acid)
Form: Capsule
Time to Take: Doesn't matter

8

WHY THE BULLETPROOF DIET WORKS FOR MEN *AND* WOMEN

igh performance is not just for men. It's also for women who want to be lean, toned, strong, and powerful; who run their own empires, raise healthy families, and will not allow their diets to destroy their performance. I want my daughter to grow up to be one of these—a Bulletproof woman. I am fortunate to have married Lana, who is such a woman and also a Karolinska Institute–trained medical doctor. When we got married, Lana was diagnosed with polycystic ovarian syndrome and was declared infertile, but we used biohacking techniques to restore her fertility and have a healthy family. Now she spends her days as a natural pregnancy and fertility consultant using Bulletproof techniques, and this experience has helped evolve specific Bulletproof Diet recommendations for women.

Men and women do have different hormone levels and different bodies, and they respond to diets quite differently as a result. Both men and women can thrive on the Bulletproof Diet, but there are some tweaks that will give women even better results.

In general, most men have no problem doing Bulletproof Intermittent Fasting, and most can learn to do any kind of intermittent fasting without Bulletproof Coffee in the morning. (But why would you want to?) However, ample anecdotal evidence in the Bulletproof online forums indicates that a significant number of women find that plain intermittent fasting causes sleeplessness, anxiety, adrenal fatigue, and an irregular menstrual cycle, among a myriad of other hormone deregulation symptoms. This makes sense from an evolutionary perspective. Women are evolved so they can remain fertile and reproduce. Even if you're not interested in having a baby, it's important to consider your fertility because one of the best indicators of your biological performance is being able to conceive and grow a healthy child. Since the Bulletproof Diet was designed to improve performance, it takes special care to boost and protect fertility in both men and women.

There are simple reasons the wrong diet has such a strong impact on women's fertility and performance. In both women and men, caloric or healthy fat restriction sends environmental signals that can impact how our genes are expressed. The science behind this is called epigenetics— the study of external forces that modify changes in gene expression—and one effect can be changes in fertility. From an epigenetic perspective, fasting or eating a low-fat diet tells our bodies, "There's a famine! Lack of food! Don't reproduce!" The female body responds much more dramatically to these signals for reasons that should be pretty obvious. Sure, it's

> While some diets can make weight loss seem so complicated, the Bulletproof Diet is simple to navigate. In the pageant world, I've seen many questionable ways for women to lose weight quickly, but the Bulletproof Diet is a healthy process. Finally I can feel good about optimizing my health while keeping the weight off and feeling better than ever. —**Erin Tjoe, Miss Hong Kong, 2014**

not ideal for men to reproduce during a famine, but they don't have to eat for two and carry the baby around. A woman simply has a much higher chance of dying during a famine if she's pregnant or nursing because of the extra demands this puts on her body.

When a woman eats too few calories, her body gets stressed in response to the famine signal and stops being fertile until food supplies (or caloric intake) return to levels that support reproduction. This is why women who are suffering from eating disorders often stop menstruating. Their bodies are in famine-panic mode and are attempting to protect the women from the stress of pregnancy by cutting off fertility.

This is one of the reasons I don't believe in calorie restriction as a generally healthy practice or advocate intense daily exercise for men or women. Many female athletes—including "weekend warriors"—also stop menstruating and are no longer fertile because it's very stressful to the body to combine extreme amounts of exercise with a low-fat, low-calorie diet. This sends a signal to your cellular epigenome that "A tiger is chasing you every single day. Your life must be under threat." Both men's and women's bodies respond to these messages with exhaustion, adrenal fatigue, and hormone problems, but women are more sensitive to these problems and feel the effects first.

I used biohacking principles to make Bulletproof Intermittent Fasting easier on the body than "traditional" intermittent fasting, allowing both women and men to realize the benefits of intermittent fasting without risking their health. Most women feel better when they avoid plain intermittent fasting and practice Bulletproof Intermittent Fasting, instead. This also hacks your gut biome to put it in fat-loss mode faster than just skipping meals because butter and especially medium-chain triglycerides suppress bad bacteria more than just not eating. Instead of going 18 hours without any calories, you get to have Bulletproof Coffee in the morning. Blended with a nice big hunk of grass-fed butter and Brain Octane Oil, this makes a satisfying breakfast for both sexes.

Instead of sending a stress signal, Bulletproof Intermittent Fasting basically tells a woman's body that it's time for autophagy (cellular cleanup) and rapid fat loss (ketosis). And it tells her gut bacteria that there's no starch, so it's time to trigger fat-burning via fasting-induced adipose factor (FIAF). Because there's no stress signal, it preserves adrenal function better than plain intermittent fasting. Since you actually use adrenal hormone epinephrine (adrenaline) that is made in your adrenal medulla to burn fat,[1] this really matters more for women than it does for men to avoid the stress signal that will cause adrenal burnout.

Making this more complex is that coffee is known to stress the adrenals. But there's also a relationship between mold toxins from coffee and adrenal dysfunction. According to research published by the World Health Organization, one of the most common mold toxins in coffee accumulates in the adrenal medulla more quickly than in any other organ except the lungs.[2, 3, 4, 5] This is a major point—mold toxins in coffee target the part of your adrenals most responsible for helping you burn fat! If you're suffering from adrenal fatigue but want to enjoy the benefits of coffee, there's a clear case to be made for choosing lab-tested coffee free from toxins that target your adrenals. Although there are no blinded studies, anecdotal reports and my own experience with adrenal fatigue recovery while enjoying Bulletproof Coffee lead me to believe that a single cup of lab-tested coffee does not interfere with adrenal recovery.

Bulletproof Coffee doesn't tell the body that you're experiencing a time of scarcity and should shut down fertility. Who ever heard of consuming delicious, satisfying grass-fed butter during a famine? Instead, it

> While on vacation in Denmark, my friend offered me coffee with butter and oil for breakfast, which sounded gross to me and not at all Danish. He dismissed me with a shrug when I called him crazy. So naturally I tried it and found it smooth and delicious. My brain turned on and my body willingly followed for several hours' touring in Copenhagen that day, something that would have usually exhausted me. My husband and I now have Bulletproof Coffee every morning without exception (including travel), and we offer it to houseguests. We get a kick out of the initial shock and horror recoil and then enjoy the reveal of energy and focus experienced by the brave who dare to try it, including our teenage nephews. **—Andrea**

I heard about Bulletproof Coffee from a colleague who spoke very highly of it. My boyfriend and I were skeptical, but we each bought a starter kit. I work for a large financial organization and have long busy days, and my boyfriend is a firefighter working various shifts. I can truly say we would never go back; we are hooked! Only one cup of Bulletproof Coffee is needed in the morning, and we no longer experience the yo-yo effect of our usual coffee. I stay focused and alert and still feel energized to head to the gym after a long day at work. **—Jennifer**

sends the message "You are in a land of plenty, with an environment full of the types of fat that make for optimally healthy babies. Be fertile! Have babies!" And the more fertile you are, the healthier your body is, and the better you will perform as a result.

The Bulletproof Diet boosts fertility not only through Bulletproof Intermittent Fasting, but also because overall it's low in sugar and high in healthy fats. It's important for women who want to get pregnant or who just need to perform at their peak to consume very little sugar. As I've already discussed, eating a lot of sugar heightens insulin levels in the body and disrupts hormone levels. Of course, proper hormone levels are key to fertility. Excess sugar also feeds yeast, which is a problem in both genders but more of a problem in women who are prone to yeast infections.

Eating plenty of high-quality fats like grass-fed butter and Brain Octane Oil also provides the extra energy that women need to sustain a pregnancy. Healthy fats are the best source of clean energy and won't lead to crashes and food cravings like sugar or carbs do. Consuming enough healthy fats will help you perform well, make your hormones work, suppress bad gut bacteria, and allow you to still lose weight. But in order to protect your fertility, it's just as important to avoid unhealthy fats as it is to eat healthy ones. Obesity is a risk factor for infertility, and synthetic trans fats can cause ovulatory infertility even in small amounts.[6]

Another way the Bulletproof Diet boosts fertility in women is by reducing inflammation. Chronic inflammation makes conception difficult, but on the Bulletproof Diet you won't be eating foods that promote inflammation like grains, dairy, and oils that are high in omega-6 fats. You may have eaten these foods in the past, though, and their effects can last up to 6 months. This is why I recommend that all women who are planning to get pregnant start the Bulletproof Diet at least 3 to 6 months before conception. Three months on the Bulletproof Diet is enough to boost your fertility, but 6 months will give your body time to clean out the harmful toxins that may have been in your previous diet while also ridding your body of chronic inflammation. The improvements you make this way can cause positive genetic changes that are inheritable by your children and even grandchildren. It's a multigenerational upgrade!

BULLETPROOF BIOHACKING TWEAKS FOR WOMEN

While the Bulletproof Diet works for men and women for all the reasons I just explained, there are a few small modifications women can make to get even better results.

ADD SALT

There is a reason that stressed women crave fatty and salty foods—adrenal exhaustion. Like with hunger, it's important not to just ignore these cravings or try to use willpower to overcome them. Remember, the adrenals produce the hormone that balances sodium and potassium levels—critical for proper cell function—so if you are stressed, consuming enough salt will help ease the burden on your already taxed adrenals. Your body is craving these foods for a reason. Listen to it. This does not mean that you should grab a bag of potato chips, as many people unfortunately do. But if you are craving fatty, salty foods, eating some delicious Bulletproof protein and veggies soaked in butter and coated with high-quality sea salt is not just a good idea—it's vital for your health. It will help you be a fierce, amazing woman who feels and looks good. And it will help you to safely practice Bulletproof Intermittent Fasting without harming your adrenals, your fertility, or your brain.

EAT PROTEIN WITH BREAKFAST

If you're over 40 and/or have significant weight to lose, it might help you in the long-term if you add some protein to your breakfast. Try mixing grass-fed collagen right into your Bulletproof Coffee. This will make you hungrier sooner than regular Bulletproof Intermittent Fasting because it kicks on your body's digestion process and effectively ends your fast, but it will also help reset your leptin levels, allowing you to both feel better in the long run and lose weight faster. When you're in maintenance mode, try adding some Bulletproof protein like pastured eggs or whey protein to your breakfast and see how you feel. Just don't eat carbs in the morning unless you want your gut bacteria to tell your body to store fat all day long!

RE-FEED CARBS

Because women's bodies are more highly attuned to stress signals, they not only really need their morning fat (and sometimes protein), but also are more carbohydrate sensitive than men. Many men thrive on the Bulletproof Diet when they have carbohydrate re-feed days only once a week. Re-feed days are days when you replenish your body with carbs by eating more of them than you normally do on the Bulletproof Diet. These carb re-feed days coincide with protein fasting days. Once a week, you'll replace the protein in your meals with healthy Bulletproof carbs. Some men perform their best when they eat carbs even less frequently. Women, however, should always re-feed with carbs at least once a week, on the day of their protein fast. Some women will need to re-feed twice a week or more once they're in maintenance mode. And having a few carbs (under 30 grams) in the evening can do wonders for women who need them.

This does not mean that you should go crazy at McDonald's! On carb re-feed days, you should stick to Bulletproof Diet principles and eat up to 300 grams of Bulletproof carbs like sweet potatoes, carrots, and white rice. This may cause you to feel a bit heavier the next day, but rest assured this is only water weight. Women who are pregnant should eat limited carbs every night while adhering to all other principles of the Bulletproof Diet. Never fast while pregnant, ever! It is extremely important for an embryo to receive adequate calories and nutrition in the womb.

MAKE IT A DECAF

If you're pregnant or actively trying to conceive, it's not a great idea to drink caffeinated coffee. Caffeine crosses the placenta, and sustained exposure to caffeine raises a fetus's heart rate. It also decreases blood flow to the placenta.[7] Lots of pregnant women have a cup of coffee every once in a while without problems, but don't drink it every day, and insist on mold-tested coffee. I recommend either replacing your Bulletproof Coffee with No-Coffee Vanilla Latte (page 254), which will give you similar results without posing any risk to your pregnancy, or switching to lab-tested decaf.

THINK ABOUT IRON

If you're following the Bulletproof Diet and eating enough red meat and organ meat, you're probably getting enough iron. But some women still need to supplement. Unfortunately, many women of childbearing age are anemic because they don't get enough red meat in their diets, and this can cause complications during pregnancy. Iron isn't one of those supplements that you want to take randomly. It's terrible for your performance to be anemic (low in iron), but taking enough iron to raise your blood ferritin level above about 75 will age you really quickly.[8] The best bet is to get your iron level tested after 2 weeks on the Bulletproof Diet to see if you need an iron supplement.

FERTILITY AND MEN

When you're thinking about starting a family, it's just as important to make sure the father is in a state of high performance and high fertility as the mother. Most men don't think that their diets have anything to do with whether or not their wife can get pregnant, but what a man does (and doesn't) eat can make a dramatic difference when it comes to his sperm quality, his fertility, and even the health of his children.

Luckily for you men, just about every aspect of the Bulletproof Diet will boost your sperm quality. One sign that you are operating in a state of high performance is that you have healthy, active sperm. The same toxins and inflammation that cause suboptimal body and brain performance also damage sperm. For men, it's best to start the Bulletproof Diet 3 months before trying to conceive, but even 30 days can make a big difference. Plus, it's more fun (and a lot more practical) to be on the Bulletproof Diet when your partner is, too!

SEX HORMONE SUPPLEMENTS FOR MEN AND WOMEN

If you want great sex hormones, whether it's for your libido or because you're planning to have a child, it's best to get your blood nutrient levels tested and check with your doctor before starting to take any supplements so that you know for sure what supplements you need. This is just as important for men as it is for women! You don't want to be shooting in the dark when it comes to sex hormones, pregnancy, and supplements. The following list of supplements will benefit most people who want to optimize their sex hormones, but it's important to know your own levels before adding them to your diet.

ZINC

This is an important supplement for male and female fertility (and thus libido), as zinc deficiency can lead to lower testosterone levels.[9] (Later in this chapter I'll explain why a woman's testosterone level is important, too.) In one study, men who took about 50 mg of elemental zinc per day for 3 months showed an improvement in sperm count, progressive motility, and fertilizing capacity.[10] They also had reduced amounts of sperm-fighting antibodies.[11]

Dose: 25 mg per day
Form: Zinc gluconate
Time to Take: With evening meal

L-ORNITHINE AND L-ARGININE

These amino acids mildly stimulate the release of human growth hormone and the formation of nitric oxide,[12] which increases blood flow, and ornithine helps to eliminate ammonia from protein digestion. L-ornithine also increases the amount of human growth hormone in the body while building muscle and reducing body fat. In women, L-arginine helps increase cervical secretions and mucus during ovulation,[13] aiding the sperm in traveling toward the egg. These amino acids are just as important for male fertility as they are for women. Due to its effect increasing blood flow, L-arginine

BULLETPROOF KIDS

When Lana and I were working to restore her fertility, we spent a lot of time researching which foods help kids grow and be healthy from before they're even conceived to when they're in the womb, and eventually throughout childhood. I found that the same foods that help adults thrive also allow kids to grow and be healthy. Once they're born, feeding children is the responsibility of both parents. I did almost all of the food preparation for my wife when she was pregnant and have done most of the cooking in our home for years. I've also helped many of my clients get their kids to be more Bulletproof, and we've found that children are at their best when they're on a high-fat diet like Bulletproof.

In general, kids who eat fewer toxins and other forms of Kryptonite like sugar and gluten behave much better than their peers. They don't melt down as frequently and are able to pay attention for longer periods of time. Keep in mind that kids do need some carbs, but incorporating some Bulletproof Diet principles into your kids' diet will help them thrive and save you the energy you may be currently wasting dealing with their tantrums. Some people worry that their kids won't survive without gluten or juice, but my kids have been following Bulletproof from a young age, and they love Bulletproof foods. Most kids naturally like butter and will eat it out of the fridge if given the opportunity, so they don't usually object to being fed a diet with more healthy fats to choose from. My kids' favorite Bulletproof dishes are sweet potato fries and creamed cauliflower with lots of grass-fed butter.

works as a natural alternative to Viagra.[14] When used for 2 weeks, it can increase sperm count and motility by 250 percent.[15] Too much L-arginine can be damaging for some people,[16] but L-ornithine regulates L-arginine levels in the body. This is why they're often packaged and used together.

Dose: 500 to 1,000 mg ornithine and 1 to 2 g arginine
Form: Capsules, separately
Time to Take: At bedtime only

ORALLY AVAILABLE GLUTATHIONE

Glutathione is an antioxidant that is made by the body and found in every cell. It guards against inflammation, toxins, free radicals, and pathogens.[17] You can think of it as your body's natural detox agent. Because it's so important for women to reduce inflammation and toxins in the body before getting pregnant, I recommend supplementing with glutathione when trying to boost fertility. Most oral supplements don't work; look for oral glutathione that has been encapsulated in MCT-based lipids along with lactoferrin to allow it to flow through the lining of the gut instead of allowing your digestion to destroy the molecules.

Dose: 100 to 200 mg
Form: Oral syringe
Time to Take: On an empty stomach at bedtime or as needed throughout the day (for erectile use!)

ACTIVATED COCONUT CHARCOAL

Like glutathione, activated coconut charcoal is a great way to detox. It literally binds toxins and removes them from your system. This is a great supplement to have on hand when you're trying to get pregnant, you're traveling, or you accidentally eat some nutritional Kryptonite. It will help you rebound a lot faster than you would otherwise. I take it whenever I travel or eat out.

Dose: 500 mg or whatever amount doesn't cause constipation

Form: Capsules

Time to Take: With suspect foods or when feeling unwell. Do not take with drugs, as they will get absorbed, too.

TESTOSTERONE IS NOT JUST FOR BODYBUILDERS

As you know, one of the most important aspects of the Bulletproof Diet is balancing hormone levels, and one hormone it focuses on increasing is testosterone. This goes for men and women. Though testosterone is usually associated with male characteristics, both men and women make testosterone and both require it in order to function properly.

Testosterone's two main jobs are to maintain libido and sexual function and to build muscle by aiding in protein synthesis. Some women worry that increasing testosterone levels in their bodies will cause them to "bulk up" and have muscles like bodybuilders, but this is impossible for women to do without an external source of testosterone. In fact, it is more common for women nowadays to produce too little testosterone, leading to weight gain, low sex drive, and a host of other symptoms. Testosterone is also needed to build healthy bones, so it is crucial for women to have the right amount of it in their bodies as they enter menopause and become at higher risk for bone fractures and osteoporosis.

So why are so many women (and even men) making too little testosterone? Unfortunately, in some of them, this is yet another consequence of eating low-fat, high-toxin, high-carb diets. When you restrict calories and/or fat, the same stress signal that shuts down fertility tells your body to begin using all of your hormone building blocks to produce cortisol instead of testosterone. Having chronically high cortisol levels can cause insulin resistance, fat gain, and the breakdown of muscle. Carbs contribute to testosterone depletion by causing blood sugar spikes. Research in men showed that the spike in blood sugar after consuming 75 g glucose is enough to lower your testosterone level by up to 25 percent for more than 2 hours.[18] In fact, both cornflakes and graham crackers were originally designed to reduce libido. At the time, sex drive was considered a "problem."

Since low-fat, high-carb diets cause our bodies to produce too little testosterone, it makes sense that a diet that is high in fat and low in sugar and carbs like the Bulletproof Diet naturally increases testosterone levels.[19] Indeed, studies have shown that male athletes who eat plenty of saturated fat, monounsaturated fat, and cholesterol had higher testosterone levels,[20] while healthy middle-aged men who ate a low-fat, high-fiber diet produced less.[21] But when it comes to increasing testosterone levels, not any fat will do. The unhealthy polyunsaturated fats that you'll avoid on the Bulletproof Diet do not increase testosterone levels the same way saturated and monounsaturated fats do.[22] The importance of testosterone is another reason that eating grass-fed, organic animal products is such a big part of the Bulletproof Diet. Dioxins, a toxin commonly found in conventionally raised animal products, have been shown to inhibit testosterone production.[23] There are fewer dioxins in organic, grass-fed meat[24] and dairy than there are in the conventional versions of these products.

After 2 weeks on the Bulletproof Diet, you will feel stronger and more vital than ever before. Whether you are a man or a woman, this is in large part because your body now has the building blocks it needs to make all of the hormones your body requires for it to thrive. I credit the Bulletproof Diet with not only the fact that I have a family at all, but also the fact that I have such healthy, bright children and a powerful, youthful Bulletproof wife!

THE BULLETPROOF DIET ROADMAP TO SWANKY NEIGHBORHOODS

It seems simple to break foods down into three categories—beneficial, neutral, and harmful—but the truth is that foods are actually far more complex than that. One of the revelations that came out of my research was that everything you eat falls somewhere on a spectrum from the most beneficial foods at one end to those that are the most harmful on the other. Some foods have slightly more to offer nutritionally than others, while some cause a bit more inflammation than others. This is where the Bulletproof Diet Roadmap comes in, a simple spectrum of foods that will guide you in making better choices for yourself, your particular body, and your unique mind. This works well for so many Bulletproof Dieters because it tells you exactly where you are on the roadmap based on what foods you're choosing and where you're headed next. With your next meal, are you heading in a solid direction or toward a less desirable area? What city is next on your roadmap and is it somewhere you really want to visit?

Once you learn the information in the roadmap, you'll be able to look at a meal and know exactly what city it's in. Depending on where you personally thrive, you'll know exactly what direction to go in. By making poor choices you can fail to lose weight on this diet (like any other), but you can't fail to stay on it because you'll always be eating somewhere on the roadmap. It's up to you to decide where you want to eat, and these chapters will give you all of the information you need to make the very best decisions.

You can use the Bulletproof Diet Roadmap here on the pages in the book, or I'll send you the full-color poster version for free when you text your name, e-mail address, and the number 122182 to 1-858-598-3980 or visit bulletproofexec.com/roadmap. I want you to learn how to navigate this roadmap so you can experience a new level of performance and energy without having to spend countless years and dollars trying to figure it all out like I did. Learning more about the beneficial and/or harmful properties of specific foods will allow you to make informed choices and give you a variety of Bulletproof options that you can continue to mix and match long after you've completed the 2-week program and are still looking great and kicking ass.

On the roadmap, foods fall into three categories along the spectrum that I've outlined in previous chapters: Bulletproof, Suspect, and Kryptonite foods. Bulletproof foods are the least-inflammatory, lowest-toxin, best choices with the highest nutritional content to supercharge your body and brain. Suspect foods have pros and cons and affect each of us differently, and Kryptonite foods have risks for everyone that far outweigh the benefits. You can—and should—train your Labrador brain to simply identify these as "not food." They're nearly certain to damage your performance and cause you to gain weight, age quickly, and lose focus.

For the next 2 weeks, you'll get amazing results from eating Bulletproof foods according to the meal plan later in the book. They'll make you feel incredibly powerful, boost your performance, help you lose weight, allow you to look younger, and improve your overall health. From there, I'll teach you how to incorporate Suspect foods (and even Kryptonite, if you choose) back into your diet and still feel (mostly) Bulletproof.

This chapter will zero in on the most important foods and the ones you'll be eating the most on the Bulletproof Diet: vegetables, fats, and proteins. These are the swanky neighborhoods because they're the ones you want to spend the most time in! In the next few chapters, the roadmap will continue to steer you through the foods you'll be eating less frequently and the spices and sweeteners you'll cook with to make the most satisfying, nutritious Bulletproof meals.

I shifted my diet to be more Bulletproof, and the results have been amazing. I lost 25 pounds without trying and while doing no cardio, though I did lift weights two or three times a week. I've also gained strength, focus, and sustained energy levels that keep me going through long 12- to 14-hour days on set. I've stopped having to worry about losing and regaining the same 5 pounds that nag me, especially when worrying about being on camera. Thanks to the Bulletproof Diet, my weight and muscle tone are as stable as my energy levels and even my emotions. Because I no longer suffer from blood sugar crashes, I don't lose my temper as easily and have far more patience both at work and at home with my 2-year-old son. But perhaps the greatest change I've noticed with the Bulletproof Diet is my ability to act on the outside like the person I always felt I was on the inside. With the extra brainpower I get from the Bulletproof Diet, I find that I'm able to communicate and express my feelings more effectively than I used to, while also having more energy to engage in social situations. I used to be content to watch from the sidelines, but now I'm more often in the center of conversations, interacting with true joy. I'm finally able to get out of my head and remain present and in the moment, where my attention, self-awareness, and performance have all dramatically improved. Losing weight, feeling amazing, and effortlessly staying in shape would have been enough. I never imagined such a simple shift in diet could provide an inner gateway to myself, but the Bulletproof Diet has done just that. **—Brandon Routh, actor**

In each section, the foods will appear in order from the ones that are most Bulletproof to those that are completely Kryptonite. Keep in mind that this is a spectrum, and that the foods are listed in order of gradually decreasing nutritional benefits and increasingly toxic contents and harmful effects. This spectrum makes the Bulletproof Diet so appealing for many of my readers because it puts you squarely in the driver's seat, giving you the power to steer your body wherever you want it to go. It's up to you to decide where on the roadmap you want to be and to make the right choices to drive yourself there.

VEGETABLES

On the Bulletproof Diet you'll be eating more vegetables than any other food. Almost all vegetables are healthy in their natural form (as long as they're not canned, fried, or otherwise tampered with), but some do have specific health benefits while others do contain harmful antinutrients, are GMOs, or have other specific properties that are likely to turn on your Labrador brain and inhibit your performance. The vegetables below appear in order from the

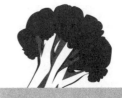

🥦 Organic Veggies

BULLETPROOF

asparagus, avocado, bok choy,* broccoli,* brussels sprouts,* cauliflower, celery, cucumber, fennel, olives

cabbage,* collards,* kale,* lettuce, radishes, spinach,* summer squash, zucchini

artichokes, butternut and winter squash, carrots, green beans, green onion, leeks, parsley

eggplant, onion, peas, peppers, shallots, tomatoes

beets, mushrooms, pumpkin, raw chard, raw collards, raw kale, raw spinach

corn (fresh on the cob)

KRYPTONITE

all other corn except fresh, canned veggies, soy

* These items should be cooked. Refer to the cooking chart for the most Bulletproof way of preparing these veggies.

Download your free color copy at http://bulletproof.com/roadmap.

most nutritious ones that are lowest in antinutrients to the ones that have the lowest amount of nutrients and the greatest risks.

BULLETPROOF VEGETABLES

AVOCADOS

A delicious plant source of monounsaturated fat, the avocado is technically a fruit, but its nutrient content makes it far more similar to a vegetable. It's one of the most Bulletproof foods you can eat. The only downside to avocados is that they're high in inflammatory omega-6 fatty acids, so if you eat a lot of them you should up your intake of omega-3s. The good news is that the omega-6 fats in avocados aren't oxidized and are solvent-free and intact, so your body can use them. If you make sure that at least half of your fat comes from saturated fat, a couple of avocados a day are fine. Just don't cook them!

OLIVES

Olives are technically a fruit, but they act more like a vegetable and should be eaten that way. Olives have been considered a "perfect food" for

CRUCIFEROUS VEGGIES AND IODINE ABSORPTION

Cruciferous veggies such as collards, Brussels sprouts, broccoli, cauliflower, cabbage, and bok choy are great Bulletproof choices, but as I discussed earlier, they're high in antinutrient oxalates that prevent nutrient absorption. Oxalates enter the body and bind with calcium ions in your blood, forming tiny crystals that can contribute to muscle weakness, pain, and possibly brain problems. Eighty percent of kidney stones are formed from oxalates. Cooking these vegetables significantly reduces these substances, so it's best to never eat these veggies raw. You can also soak them in lemon juice or use a Bulletproof technique called calcium loading by adding a calcium capsule to the cooking water. The calcium reacts with the oxalic acid, rendering it harmless.

centuries, and for good reason. There are very few toxins in olives, and they're one of the safer plant sources of fat. Just watch out for olives packed in bad oils or flavored with hidden MSG.

BOK CHOY

Also known as Chinese cabbage, bok choy has almost zero calories and carbs and very little flavor. I think it's a great platform for delicious grass-fed butter. Just make sure to cook it.

BRUSSELS SPROUTS

Brussels sprouts have potent anticancer compounds that assist in DNA repair. They're also high in potassium, folate, vitamin C, calcium, fiber, and iron; low in calories and carbs; have a low toxin load; and are easy to prepare. Like all cruciferous vegetables, they're not suitable raw.

COLLARDS

Collard greens and other cruciferous vegetables contain 3,3′-diindolyl-methane, which modulates immune function and protects against bacteria, cancer, and viruses.

SPINACH

Popeye knew something about nutrition. Plus, he was ripped! Spinach is low in carbs and calories and extremely high in carotenoids, folate, vitamin C, calcium, iron, and vitamin K_1. Just remember to cook your spinach.

KALE

Kale is high in beta-carotene, vitamin K_1, vitamin C, lutein, and zeaxanthin and has a moderate amount of calcium. Kale also contains a potent anticarcinogen called sulforaphane, which works with glutathione to remove toxins from human cells.[1] Just say no to raw kale salads—like all vegetables that are high in oxalates, kale is best cooked.

ASPARAGUS

Asparagus is fairly low in carbs and calories but packs a ton of nutrition. It's high in vitamin K_1, iron, thiamine, and riboflavin, and also has a modest amount of soluble fiber to nourish your gut bacteria.

BROCCOLI

Broccoli is high in vitamin C, fiber, phosphorus, calcium, folate, vitamin K_1, carotenoids, and has some unique health-promoting compounds like diindolylmethane, which has antiviral, anticancer, and antibacterial properties.[2] Men who eat large amounts of broccoli also have a reduced risk of prostate cancer.[3]

CABBAGE

Cabbage is low in carbs and antinutrients and high in potassium, calcium, and vitamin K_1, but it is also likely to be high in pesticides, so it's a good idea to buy organic. It is cruciferous, so limit raw cabbage or try fermenting it and see if that agrees with you. Sauerkraut and kimchi are two popular forms of fermented cabbage.

CAULIFLOWER

Cauliflower is low in carbs and calories but high in vitamin C, potassium, calcium, and fiber and has a moderate amount of vitamin K_1. Cauliflower also has sulforaphane, glucosinolates, carotenoids, and indole-3-carbinol, a compound that helps repair DNA and fights cancer.

CELERY

Celery has a small amount of calcium, potassium, folate, beta-carotene, and sodium; a decent amount of fiber; almost no calories; and a very mild flavor that makes it very versatile. The Environmental Working Group found 13 different pesticides when testing celery,[4] so it's a good idea to go organic.

CUCUMBER

Cucumbers are high in potassium, phosphorus, fiber, and not much else. Try them dipped in guacamole or blended into salad dressings for a boost in flavor and nutrition. You can eat as much cucumber as you like without worrying!

DARK GREEN LEAFY LETTUCE

Dark varieties of lettuce like arugula, escarole, and mâche are high in potassium, carotenoids, vitamin K_1, iron, and fiber, but rot very easily and get moldy. Try to buy organic lettuce whenever possible and eat it when it's fresh.

RADISHES

Radishes are high in vitamin C, folate, fiber, and calcium. They're low in toxins and are more protected from pesticides than most vegetables because they grow underground.

SUMMER SQUASHES

Technically fruits, squashes are so low in sugar that most people consider them vegetables. They're a great source of potassium, fiber, and, if you need some, carbs. Squash is low in toxins other than the pesticides they're usually sprayed with. Make sure to wash them thoroughly.

ZUCCHINI

This summer squash tastes great raw or cooked; is high in potassium, phosphorus, and fiber; and is low in carbs. Watch out for genetically modified zucchini, which is unfortunately common.

SUSPECT VEGETABLES

ARTICHOKES

Artichokes are low in toxins other than some acids that are present in the raw plant and a very small amount of the toxin found in nightshades. If you know you're nightshade sensitive, try to avoid artichokes.

GREEN BEANS

Green beans are high in calcium, iron, potassium, fiber, and carotenoids. They're fairly low in antinutrients and usually aren't GMO, but are suspect because they cause digestive problems in some people due to their lectin content. They're harder on the gut if you eat them raw.

EGGPLANT

Eggplants are low in toxins and high in potassium, phosphorus, and fiber, but they're a nightshade vegetable. If you can tolerate them, they absorb grass-fed butter like nothing else.

PEPPERS

Peppers are higher in vitamin C than oranges and contain lots of potassium, phosphorus, folate, lycopene, and carotene. Dried peppers or peppers that aren't super fresh have a particularly strong risk of mold toxin contamination. These are in the nightshade family, as well.

TOMATOES

Tomatoes are high in beta-carotene, lycopene, and folate. They're also high in phosphorus and potassium, but do contain some fructose and are a nightshade vegetable. Tomatoes are also fairly high in histamines, so pay attention if you feel hungry, tired, or cranky after eating them.

GARLIC

Garlic feeds healthy gut bacteria and is reported to have antifungal effects. So why would I recommend mostly avoiding such a tasty miracle herb? This is one of the most controversial and unpopular recommendations I make, but it's because garlic has psychoactive effects. I first became aware of this during 40 Years of Zen brain training, where I learned advanced meditation states. The trainer cautioned me to avoid garlic or the brain training wouldn't work as well. I was skeptical, and after I'd learned what my brain

NIGHTSHADE VEGETABLES

Nightshades are a category of plants including foods, herbs, shrubs, and trees. Tobacco and belladonna, a plant with poisonous berries, are both nightshades, and several popular vegetables also fall into this category, including eggplant, potatoes, tomatoes, sweet and hot peppers, tomatillos, pimentos, and cayenne peppers. These foods all contain two possible sources of Kryptonite. The first is a group of substances called alkaloids, which can impact nerves, muscles, joints, and digestive function in some people.[5] There's cause for concern that nightshade alkaloids can contribute to loss of calcium from bones and deposit that calcium in soft tissue, because nightshades contain calcitriol, a hormone thousands of times stronger than vitamin D.[6] The second issue with nightshades, as I discussed earlier, is the presence of antinutrient lectins, which can cause autoimmune reactions independent of the alkaloid problem.

There are some of us who can eat nightshade vegetables with few obvious problems and others who are more sensitive or have autoimmune reactions to them. This makes all nightshade foods Suspect. One thing to keep in mind is that cooking lowers alkaloid levels in nightshade vegetables by about half. This means it's safest to always cook these vegetables even if you aren't particularly sensitive to them. If you are sensitive, you should avoid them altogether.

If you're not sure, eat a ton of nightshades for a day—salsa, peppers, eggplants, potatoes—and see how you feel for the next 3 days. You may be surprised.

could do at the end of my first week, I ate some garlic and tried to meditate a while later. My brain didn't work the same way. It was much more difficult for me to focus, and it took 4 days for me to get back in the zone.

I did some research and learned that religious leaders in history knew the dark side of garlic. In one story from Islam, when Satan left the Garden of Eden garlic sprang from his first cloven hoofprint and onions from the second. In Jainism, garlic and onions are strictly forbidden because of their disturbing effect on the mind. Hindu and Buddhist teachings in

Nepal and Tibet assert that garlic creates agitation and aggression, interferes with focus, and makes it difficult to reach higher spiritual states. These obviously aren't scientific sources, but they support my observation.

Some of the most interesting information about garlic comes from one of the pioneers of electroencephalography (EEG) neurofeedback, Robert C. Beck. He's admittedly a controversial figure and not all of his inventions worked, but he created some solid protocols for his time. Beck researched the effects of garlic on brain function after being told it slowed reaction time when he was a military pilot in the 1950s. In the 1970s, he ran an EEG manufacturing company and found that people showed far less brain activity after eating garlic and that their brains waves had become desynchronized.[7]

In several different studies, higher-dose or longer-term use of garlic has also been shown to cause a number of other health problems, such as liver stress and inflammation.[8] The most convincing evidence for me is that garlic breaks my meditation, and it is harder for me to focus when I eat garlic prior to meditating. Don't get me wrong; garlic is great medicinally for certain conditions, but it should not be a staple additive to food for people who want to be in charge of their brains. Eat it when you're sick and don't need to focus very well!

ONIONS

Onions are in the same family as garlic and share a similar chemistry. If you're training your brain or meditating heavily, you should avoid them entirely, but they appear to have less of an impact than garlic. You should test them out to see how they affect you personally. I use them occasionally as a flavoring agent but don't recommend eating them daily. They're also pretty high in sugar, so limit them to dinner. Salad onions have much less of an effect, so I usually use those.

BEETS

Beets are low in antinutrients except oxalates and high in potassium, sodium, phosphorus, fiber, and folate, but they can be a sneaky source of unwanted carbs due to their high sugar content. They may also be genetically modified. The USDA has been sued in the past for encouraging and allowing farmers to plant GMO sugar beets, and GMO beets may spread their pollen to other types of beets.

PEAS

Like green beans, many varieties of peas often contain antinutrient lectins that cause digestive problems, but many people report these issues as being worse with peas than they are with green beans. Peas are very high in starchy carbs, so if they agree with you they're best limited to the evening.

KRYPTONITE VEGETABLES

MUSHROOMS

This is another time when I don't like what I'm writing, but it's the truth. Mushrooms are wonderful medical fungi, but we haven't studied thousands of the chemicals in commonly eaten mushrooms. There are definitely health arguments for eating medicinal mushrooms, as they are believed to boost your immune system. But mushrooms also encourage the growth of yeast in the body. White button mushrooms (*Agaricus bisporus*) contain p-hydrazinobenzoic acid, which is implicated in smooth vascular cell proliferation, which is part of how your blood vessels remodel themselves after injury. This is a sign of muscular injury and is not a positive thing for vascular health. Even though mushrooms have been used as a tasty food source for years, there is a hidden downside and there are better choices. It's like taking medicine you don't really need. Since mushrooms can be a mixed bag, I recommend limiting your exposure during the 2-week program. Then see an herbalist if you want to use medicinal mushrooms like reishi, shiitake, etc.

ALL CANNED VEGETABLES

Canned vegetables are usually contaminated with bisphenol A (BPA), from the canning process and are often high in histamines.[9] BPA is used to make plastics and exhibits hormonelike properties in the body. To top it off, preservatives and other additives are often mixed with the vegetables to increase their shelf life, while heating them to high temperatures lowers their nutrient levels. If fresh veggies aren't an option, there's no reason you can't heat up some frozen vegetables, instead. Frozen vegetables are far superior to canned because they are normally picked and frozen at the peak of freshness and aren't tampered with like canned vegetables are.

FATS

It may seem counterintuitive at first to make fats the core of the Bulletproof Diet, but given how much your body needs them, it makes sense. Eating a lot of healthy fats is actually much better for you than eating high amounts of almost any other type of food. Excessive sugar and protein are particularly harmful. In the past few decades, the trend has been to replace fats with sugar, but this has proven to be terrible for our health. As you read earlier, replacing carbs with too much protein can be hard on the liver as it struggles to break down all the amino acids in the protein. The macronutrient that burns the most

Oil & Fats

BULLETPROOF ▲

Bulletproof Brain Octane Oil, Bulletproof XCT Oil, Bulletproof Ghee, Bulletproof Chocolate, Bulletproof Cocoa Butter, pastured egg yolks,† krill oil, grass-fed red meat fat and marrow, avocado oil, coconut oil, sunflower lecithin

fish oil, grass-fed butter and ghee

palm oil, palm kernel, pastured bacon fat, raw macadamias, extra virgin olive oil

raw almonds, hazelnuts, walnuts, cashew butter, non-GMO soy lecithin

duck and goose fat, grain-fed butter and ghee

factory chicken fat, safflower, sunflower, canola, peanut, soy cottonseed, corn, and vegetable oils, heated nuts and oils, flaxseed oil

KRYPTONITE ▼

margarine and other artificial trans fats, oils made from GMO grains, commercial lard

† Verify that you are not allergic to eggs.

Download your free color copy at http://bulletproof.com/roadmap.

cleanly and contains the most energy is fats, particularly the healthiest, most Bulletproof fats listed here in order from the most nutrient dense to those that are nutritionally void, toxic Kryptonite.

BULLETPROOF FATS

GRASS-FED ANIMAL FAT (BONE MARROW, TALLOW, LARD, ETC., BUT NOT POULTRY FAT)

These fats are high in nutrients, essential fatty acids, protein, minerals, antioxidants, and fat-soluble nutrients that are hard to get elsewhere. Bone marrow is especially high in omega-3 fats, and some researchers believe that cracking open scavenged bones and consuming the marrow was what allowed humans to develop large brains. These are *the* most Bulletproof sources of fats on earth! Remember that as long as they're grass-fed, cows are plant based.

GRASS-FED BUTTER

Butter from grass-fed animals is high in fat-soluble vitamins, antioxidants, healthy fats, and vitamins A, E, D, and K. Grain feeding causes a massive drop in all the beneficial compounds in butter, introduces new toxins, and raises omega-6 levels. It's crucial to choose grass-fed butter every time.

GRASS-FED GHEE

Ghee has all the micronutrients and antioxidants of butter, but it goes through one more step of processing that makes is just a little more Bulletproof. Cultured grass-fed butter is heated for a short period of time to remove the water, the milk protein called casein, and lactose. The final product is even more nutrient dense than butter without the casein and lactose that can be irritating to some people. For those who are especially sensitive to dairy or who have gut damage, ghee is a must.

VIRGIN COCONUT OIL

Virgin coconut oil has more saturated fat than almost any other food, making it a good choice for cooking because it's so stable. If you can eat enough of it, the small amount of real MCT in coconut oil can boost brain function, increase ketone formation, and assist in fat loss. Beware of copra oil, a type of coconut oil that is particularly moldy.

MCT OIL

This is a liquid coconut extract that is a mixture of medium- and short-chain fats. MCT oil also promotes ketone formation and brain functionality even better than coconut oil.

BRAIN OCTANE OIL AND XCT OIL

Brain Octane Oil is a staple of the Bulletproof Diet and a key ingredient in Bulletproof Coffee. It's made purely of C8 MCTs, the cleanest, most potent MCT, proven four times as effective as coconut oil at raising ketones. Brain Octane converts to ketones within minutes, making it a powerful tool to suppress hunger and fuel your brain in a way that other MCTs do not. It's also flavorless, odorless, and easier on your stomach than most other MCTs.

XCT Oil is a blend of two MCTs—C8 and C10. XCT is slightly less potent at converting to ketones than Brain Octane, but you'll still get the mental and metabolic boost.

Some MCT manufacturers produce products using solvents like hexane, which can leave behind chemical residues. Brain Octane Oil and

I started taking Brain Octane Oil about 2 years ago and recently managed to get to the strongest form of MCT, which I use in my Bulletproof Coffee every day. Besides going back to college at 65 and getting straight As, I've also been almost completely healed from lifetime, chronic asthma after going Bulletproof. I don't get sick with coughs or colds now. This has changed my life! Another amazing thing that happened after going Bulletproof is that I weaned myself off of blood pressure meds. I check my blood pressure regularly and all is well. Thanks again. **—Charlotte**

XCT Oil are cleaned with activated charcoal and refined without the toxic chemicals. Neither contains lauric acid (C12), the cheapest and least potent MCT in coconut oil.

FISH/KRILL OILS

These beneficial omega-3 fatty acids improve cardiovascular health, fight inflammation, improve brain function, and reduce your risk of cancer. It's important to choose a high-quality brand, as the cheaper ones may be oxidized during processing. Krill oil comes packaged with astaxanthin, a potent antioxidant that may help reduce oxidation during processing. As I mentioned earlier, these oils can also help improve sleep quality. I prefer krill oil for that purpose.

FERMENTED COD LIVER OIL (FCLO)

Cod liver oil is one of the most nutrient-dense substances on earth. By weight it's the richest source of fat-soluble vitamins, plus it's high in antioxidants, minerals, and fatty acids. Unfortunately, modern methods of producing cod liver oil produce extreme amounts of vitamin A, and the distillation process removes other nutrients and cofactors. Luckily, Green Pasture ferments their cod liver oil using a traditional process that retains all the beneficial effects. They also test their cod liver oil for contaminants, heavy metals, and even mold. They are the only brand that does this.

NON-GMO SOY LECITHIN OR SUNFLOWER LECITHIN

Lecithin, almost the only part of the soy plant worth eating, is an important nutrient for brain performance and overall health. (Note this is lecithin the protein, not the antinutrient food toxin lectin or the satiation hormone leptin.) Some people experience a mental boost from consuming lecithin, probably because it raises the level of an excitatory neurotransmitter called acetylcholine. There is some evidence that a small amount of soy phytoestrogen can be present in some lecithin brands, but not enough for me (or you) to be concerned about.

CACAO BUTTER

Cocoa butter and cacao butter are the same thing, but most companies use the term cocoa butter when marketing skin-care products. Make sure you're buying something that is meant to be eaten. Cacao butter is a plant fat that is high in saturated and monounsaturated fat, and its polyphenols and antioxidants can improve cardiovascular health and regulate healthy blood pressure. It adds an incredibly rich chocolate aftertaste to foods. Some people add it to their Bulletproof Coffee, or you can melt it and use it in any type of dessert recipe. It's an amazing way of adding a chocolate flavor to foods without actually adding chocolate. I've even added it to fish dishes to make a delicious, rich mole flavor. Quality matters greatly when it comes to cacao butter, as this is generally one of the moldiest types of fats you can get. Look for single-estate brands.

AVOCADO OIL

Avocado oil is great in small amounts, but it's best to eat avocados to get it. Too much extracted oil can exceed the Bulletproof limit of polyunsaturated fats. Even though it has a high flash point, it's not a good idea to use it for cooking because it oxidizes easily, and there is a risk of solvents being used in its manufacture. Stick to reputable brands!

SUSPECT FATS

EXTRA VIRGIN OLIVE OIL

Some people consider olive oil a panacea, but it's on the Suspect list because of its high omega-6 content, and because 69 percent of olive oil in a recent survey contained other oils that weren't on the label.[10] Because it's so prone to oxidation, olive oil should never be cooked. Choose high-quality brands that are packaged in dark glass to avoid oxidation. Purity of olive oil is extremely important, as many commercial brands contain canola and/or other Kryptonite oils. Use it on salads in moderation if it agrees with you. I mix ⅔ Brain Octane Oil oil with ⅓ olive oil to achieve the same flavor with less polyunsaturated oil.

PALM AND PALM KERNEL OIL

Cold processed palm oil is a good source of fat, but it shouldn't be consumed in large amounts. It's high in polyunsaturated fat, plus palmitic acid is shown to escort a bacterial gut toxin called lipopolysaccharide (LPS) into the liver. MCTs actually protect the liver from the same toxin, which is why it's a Bulletproof choice. Palm kernel oil, which comes from the nut of the same tree, contains less polyunsaturated fat and is more heat stable. It's also higher in medium-chain fats and overall is a better option than regular palm oil.

UNHEATED NUT OILS (MACADAMIA, ALMOND, WALNUT, ETC.)

Nut oils are mostly made of monounsaturated and polyunsaturated fatty acids that are prone to oxidation when exposed to air, light, and heat. When inside nuts, these oils are relatively stable, but when extracted, they're defenseless. These oils should be stored in the fridge and never heated, but heating is often part of the extraction process and it's hard to find ones that are cold pressed. Of these, macadamia and almond oils are the best choices, as they are the highest in monounsaturated and saturated fats.

PASTURED BACON

Pastured bacon is high in nutrients, healthy fats, and antioxidants but also has somewhat high levels of omega-6 fats and a real potential for toxins and pathogens. I love bacon, so I stock up on pork bellies from pastured, heritage-breed hogs in the fall and then baconify them by curing the meat myself—problem solved in a most delicious way! Factory-farmed pork and bacon fat are likely to have antibiotic and mold-toxin residues.

GRAIN-FED BUTTER AND GHEE

When dairy cows are fed grains, they become sick, malnourished, and weak. They're often injected with hormones and antibiotics to increase milk production, but the milk that comes out has fewer nutrients and traces of those hormones and antibiotics in it. Grain-fed butter and ghee are more likely to be contaminated with mold and other toxins because mold is a major issue in agricultural feed, and it bioaccumulates in animal milk. Sixty percent of mold toxin accumulates in the casein, so eating only the fat is safer than drinking milk from these animals. Bottom line—these won't harm you in a pinch, but they won't provide nearly the same benefits as the grass-fed versions.

PASTURED DUCK AND GOOSE FAT

These fats are high in nutrients and brain-boosting cholesterol. Duck and goose fat are more resistant to oxidation than chicken fat, but less so than beef and lamb. It's just about impossible to find pastured fats like these except at gourmet stores or hunting lodges—if you find them, stock up!

PASTURED CHICKEN FAT

Chicken skin is a good source of collagen protein, but the skin also has the most fat in it, much of which is inflammatory omega-6 linoleic acid. It's okay to consume chicken fat every now and then, but you should only eat the skin on pastured chickens if it's not burned or grilled. Denatured protein mixed with oxidized omega-6 fat (think: buffalo wings) is not Bulletproof.

KRYPTONITE FATS AND OILS

SAFFLOWER AND SUNFLOWER OILS

Safflower seeds are heated to high temperatures to extract the oil, but this makes the fragile oils oxidize. Sunflower oil has the same problem, but is even more prone to oxidation than safflower oil and it has a lower smoke point. This pretty much guarantees that the sunflower oil you eat is oxidized. Eating a handful of sunflower seeds on occasion is far more natural, assuming you can tolerate them!

COMMERCIAL LARD

Grain-fed cattle are fed contaminated grains, forced to live in unsanitary conditions, and injected with antibiotics and synthetic hormones. The toxins and pathogens from their environment are collected in their fat tissue. When you consume commercial lard, you're eating this toxic mixture. Commercial lard is also extremely low in nutrients and healthy fats compared to its grass-fed counterpart. It's usually hydrogenated, too.

CANOLA, CORN, COTTONSEED, FLAX, PEANUT, SOY, AND OTHER "VEGETABLE" OILS

As you read in Chapter 3, there is nothing to gain from consuming these oils, and they can be damaging to your health in the short and long term even in small amounts. Avoid as much as possible.

MARGARINE AND OTHER ARTIFICIAL TRANS FATS

If you could pick one type of fat that would destroy your performance, decrease your brain function, damage your health, and shorten your life, it would have to be this. They lower your HDL cholesterol and increase your risk of heart disease, increase your triglyceride levels, and damage your arteries and your heart. These fats are especially bad for brain function, as they cause inflammation in your brain. Artificial trans fats have been linked to cancer, dementia, Alzheimer's disease, liver damage, infertility, and depression. Trans fats are usually made from GMO grain, legume, and seed oils, so there's the added health risk of genetic modification. Many countries have begun to crack down on trans fats, but they're still found in tons of products. Some companies have cleverly hidden them in their ingredient lists by making their portion sizes just small enough to legally be labeled trans fat–free.

PROTEINS

Protein is extremely important because it provides the building blocks for your muscles. That doesn't mean that you should eat as much protein as possible, however. What it does mean is that you should focus on eating moderate amounts of the highest-quality protein you can find. As you read in Chapter 3, a good general rule is to eat between 0.325 and 0.75 gram of protein a day per pound of body weight. Eating a moderate-protein diet is also going to provide the best antiaging benefits. By following the Bulletproof Diet, you should be in a position to build muscle and shed fat, but you can use these principles to be a bodybuilder by simply upping the protein amount. Because protein builds muscle, bodybuilders need more protein than this, but it comes at a metabolic cost. However, these general guidelines are for people who want to live a healthy life and look good while doing it.

BULLETPROOF PROTEINS

GRASS-FED BEEF AND LAMB

Grass-fed beef and lamb are two of the best sources of protein on the Bulletproof Diet, but be aware that grass-fed cattle are often fed grain for 30 days before slaughter to get the animal fat. This removes the health benefits, so insist on grass-fed and grass-*finished*, which means the animal only ate grass!

PASTURED EGGS

An increasing number of people are allergic to eggs but don't know they have the allergy. Only eat eggs during the 2-week program if you are certain you're not allergic. Except for potassium and some amino acids, most of the nutrients in eggs are in the yolks,

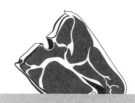

Protein

BULLETPROOF

Bulletproof Whey, Bulletproof Collagen Protein, Bulletproof CollaGelatin, grass-fed beef and lamb, pastured eggs† and gelatin, colostrum

low-mercury wild fish such as anchovies, haddock, petrale sole, sardines, sockeye salmon, summer flounder, trout

pastured pork, clean whey isolate,* pastured duck and goose

factory farmed eggs,† pastured chicken and turkey

heated whey, hemp protein, factory-farmed meat

high-mercury or farmed seafood, rice and pea protein

KRYPTONITE

soy protein, wheat protein, beans, cheese and other pasteurized or cooked dairy (except butter)

* Whey protein should be cold processed and cross-flow microfiltered (CFM). People who are sensitive to dairy should use isolate over concentrate.

Download your free color copy at http://bulletproof.com/roadmap.

which are extremely high in micronutrients. This means egg-white omelets are not Bulletproof! Just like butter, egg yolks lose most of their nutritional benefits when they come from an animal that was fed antibiotics and GMO corn and soy, which is the diet of essentially all chicken you'll find in supermarkets.

Pastured egg yolks have a deep-golden color from the vitamin A and antioxidants, while grain-fed eggs look like regular grain-fed butter—pale and watery. *Mother Earth News* magazine tested the nutritional value of pastured eggs from 14 farms and compared them to industrial eggs. In the pastured eggs, they found seven times more beta-carotene, three times more vitamin E, two-thirds more vitamin A, and two times more omega-3s.[11] This is serious—if you want to perform well and look good, it's your job to eat foods with the highest nutrition density you can find. Which egg would you choose?

GRASS-FED COLLAGEN PROTEIN

Consuming collagen balances your amino acid ratios, and gut bacteria can turn collagen into butyric acid, which is very good for your gut. Collagen also heals cartilage and supports tissue repair, allowing you to have youthful, flexible joints and wrinkle-free skin. It also supports the matrix of your bones and the lining of your arteries.[12] Collagen is largely missing from modern diets. The cheapest but least convenient way to get collagen is the way your grandmother did, by making bone broth by boiling bones from grass-fed animals. Instead, I use collagen from grass-fed cows, which is predigested with enzymes to make it easier to absorb than your other option, which is gelatin from grass-fed cows. Most gelatin on the market comes from industrial animals and is derived from heat processing instead of enzyme processing and doesn't provide the same benefits as grass-fed, enzymatically processed, enzymatically hydrolyzed collagen.

COLOSTRUM

Colostrum is the first kind of milk produced by cows to support their babies. It's loaded with immune-stimulating compounds and growth factors that will protect you from pathogens and has been shown to help prevent intestinal injury and decrease intestinal permeability. It's available as a powder protein supplement. Make sure yours comes from grass-fed cows.

WHEY PROTEIN CONCENTRATE

Whey protein works in the liver to increase your levels of the antioxidant glutathione because quality whey contains all the key amino acids for glutathione production. Whey is commonly used to increase muscle mass in bodybuilders and in the elderly. The only problem is that whey protein is processed in ways that can make it quite inflammatory. I recommend 2 tablespoons per day at most, unless you're working out a lot, in which case up to 4 tablespoons per day is worthwhile. If you rely on whey protein for more of your daily protein requirement, you end up getting excessive amounts of the amino acids cysteine and methionine, which can be inflammatory in excessive amounts. If you want more protein powder, I suggest adding grass-fed collagen protein to your whey to balance out the amino acid ratios.

WILD-CAUGHT SEAFOOD

Wild-caught seafood is high in healthy fats, micronutrients, microminerals, and antioxidants. All fish have some mercury, and there is considerable debate about how dangerous it is given that it comes with selenium, which can be protective.[13] The evidence is still out, but based on my experience I believe mercury in fish does have a negative impact. After I lost the100 pounds of fat, I dedicated myself to a yoga practice so I could learn how to use my newly found nonobese body. One of the ways I tracked my process was to stand on one leg with my eyes closed during yoga class (tree pose). It's surprisingly difficult to do this, but I learned to stay upright for 20 to 30 seconds by taking advantage of very small changes in my posture, ones I could barely feel. In some classes, though, I'd tip over after only 2 to 3 seconds no matter how hard I tried. For about 6 months I tried to figure out what the variable was, and I discovered that my balance was impacted when I had sushi for dinner the day before a yoga class.

This is not a terrible surprise in retrospect. Neurotoxins from foods and our environment are known to have subtle impact on our nervous systems. Mercury is a documented cause of ototoxicity, where there can be damage to the nerves in the ear. A Japanese study found balance system problems in 14 people after exposure to organic mercury.[14] We also know that some people who have more mercury in their systems are more sensitive to problems with candida and other yeast in the gut.[15] When I had trouble balancing in yoga class, I had my urinary mercury levels tested, and they were high, indicating that my body burden of mercury was, too. This is why I believe the safest choice is to choose fish that are lowest in mercury, which are:

- Anchovies
- Haddock
- Petrel sole
- Sardines

- Sockeye salmon
- Summer flounder
- Wild tilapia
- Wild trout

SUSPECT PROTEINS

POULTRY

As a general rule, it's okay to have pork, duck, goose, chicken, or turkey a few times per week, but you'll benefit less than you would from sticking with fish or grass-fed ruminants. One of the problems with poultry is that poultry fat is high in omega-6 fats. In addition, the vast majority of chickens you can buy (even organic ones) are fed corn and soy. This means the fats are even lower in quality than they naturally would be and tend to contain more toxins than you'd find in grass-fed animals. It's incredibly hard to find good-quality chicken. If you can find pastured organic chicken from a local farmer, it will be a big step in the right direction, but the fat will still be lower in quality than grass-fed beef or lamb because of the high omega-6 content.

PASTURED PORK

Pigs will eat just about anything, and most farmers give their pigs grain that is often tainted with mold toxins. Pigs are very sensitive to mold toxins; humans are the only animals who are even more sensitive. Large industrial operators are aware of how mold toxins impact weight gain in pigs and feed cheaper, moldier feed before slaughter to fatten them up. When pigs eat mold toxins, the toxins collect in their fat tissue. Pigs slaughtered during winter or spring tend to have more toxins stored in their fat because the foods they eat in winter are stored in silos where mold grows. Summer and fall pigs eat fresh food that hasn't had time to degrade. Finally, pork tends to be higher in histamine—if you feel tired or dizzy or get an allergy attack after eating it, you may have eaten pork that was stored too long before cooking, giving the proteins time to break down.

PASTURED DUCK, GOOSE, CHICKEN, AND TURKEY

Birds are one of the few animals that naturally eat grains. For this reason and because they're often fed supplemental corn and soy, ducks and geese are higher in omega-6 fats than many other types of meat even if they're pastured. Chickens and turkeys eat even more grains than ducks and geese, so they're more likely to be exposed to mold toxins.

FACTORY-FARMED EGGS

Factory-raised chickens are forced to eat low-quality grains their entire lives and are fed antibiotics. Luckily, evolution has worked hard to prevent the baby chicks from being damaged by their moms' diet. The mother hens will filter out and collect many of the toxins that would normally be present in the eggs. This means the eggs of factory-farmed hens are fairly low in toxins, but they're also much lower in nutrients than pastured eggs.

CLEAN WHEY PROTEIN ISOLATE

Whey protein isolate is a highly processed and refined version of whey protein. Heating it to a high temperature denatures the protein structures and destroys the glutathione-boosting properties of whey protein. It also oxidizes the small amount of fat that's still in the whey. Whey protein isolate is also lower in nutrients and growth factors than whey concentrate. However, this is a good option for people who are sensitive to lactose and/or the small amounts of casein in whey protein concentrate.

SPROUTED LEGUMES

Whether or not you tolerate beans depends largely on how they're prepared, your genetics, your allergies, and your gut biome. Sprouted and/or soaked legumes are the healthiest, as the nutrients are still available and the process makes antinutrients less potent. But legumes still contain allergens and digestive inhibitors, and it's not unusual for them to have mold toxins,[16] so look for high-quality ones. Garbanzo beans (chickpeas) are a popular legume, but the problem with chickpeas is that they're one of the most allergenic legumes,[17] almost on par with peanuts. They're a source of fairly low-nutrient carbs and low-quality protein with a high risk for inflammation and allergic reactions. Screw hummus. Eat guacamole, instead.

KRYPTONITE PROTEINS

FARMED SEAFOOD

Farmed seafood is high in pesticides, toxins, heavy metals, parasites, pathogens, and environmental contaminants. It's also much lower in nutrients and healthy fats than wild-caught seafood, and Norwegian salmon farms are starting to impact healthy wild fish populations around the world. Fish farming in the open ocean is not sustainable, kills wild fish, and causes pollution, and the food it makes doesn't lead you to a state of high performance. Steer clear of foods that are harmful not only to you, but to the entire planet!

FACTORY-FARMED MEAT

Animals in factory farms are fed whatever will cost the least to make them fat, including contaminated grains, garbage, stale junk food, and leftover animal parts like chicken beaks and feathers. Because these animals live in such horrible conditions, they're pumped full of antibiotics to keep them alive long enough to last until slaughter. The antibiotics, hormones, and synthetic estrogen compounds these cows are given also make them fatter. In addition, feedlot animals are far lower in nutrients than grass-fed animals. If you can't find, afford, or bring yourself to buy grass-fed meat, choose the leanest cuts possible to avoid the toxins that accumulate in the fats and supplement with fish or krill oil to get more of the fat you need.

SOY

Soy milk and soy protein have been sold as health foods, but they're not. In fact, soy is Kryptonite for several reasons. Soy crops may have fewer problems with mold toxin contamination than corn or grains, but it is still a significant issue. Since almost all of the fat in soy is from polyunsaturated omega-6s and is treated at high heat when processed, you're almost guaranteed to be consuming oxidized fats if you eat soy. Soybeans contain many of the antinutrients I already discussed, and the proteins in soy, especially GMO soy, are also extremely allergenic. This is especially problematic because soy is almost always GMO, unless it's labeled "organic."[18] It is well known that soy inhibits thyroid function, which over time will make you slow and fat because it slows down your metabolism. But one of the biggest problems with soy is the phytoestrogen content. Soy contains plant isoflavones that mimic estrogen in humans. This leads to hormonal problems and may increase your risk of cancer.

People like to tout the health benefits of soy by using the high-soy diets in Asia as an example, but Asians actually consume far less soy than many people think. This is because they do not use soy as a meat or dairy replacement. If you drink one glass of soy milk or eat one soy burger, you're consuming far more soy protein than the average Japanese person, who only eats about 8 grams of soy a day. Fermented soy, which is commonly found in Asian cuisine, is quite different than regular soy because the fermentation process reduces the amount of antinutrients in products such as tempeh, miso, natto, and soy sauce. But these products still contain

Vexed at having antacids pushed my way by my doctor for a problem I knew was not heartburn, I took my health into my own hands. The pains were frightening. I could feel my body begging me to change. I determined that the main (but not sole) contributing factor to my constant chest pain was the medication I depended on for years to drive my productivity. I was not prepared for the loss of productivity that followed. Conforming my diet to the scientifically backed Bulletproof parameters was essential to the process of regaining control of my mind and keeping the pain at bay. I've ramped back up to my former productivity, and now I'm growing professionally and feel myself truly living. **—Antonio**

high levels of biogenic amines like histamine, fungal metabolites, natural and added MSG,[19] and GMO ingredients (unless labeled "organic").

BEANS

Beans have been touted as a health food, but they actually disturb digestion, impair stomach acid production, retard growth, and contain fiber, lectins, and digestive inhibitors that can hurt your gut.[20] Beans lose a lot of their nutrients when cooked (and the phytates they contain prevent minerals from being absorbed) and are almost as high in carbs as pasta. Cooking alone often isn't enough to stop beans from causing severe digestive upset (and usually flatulence), but you can remove many of the lectins by properly soaking, rinsing, fermenting, and then cooking beans. Beans do have some resistant starch, which may be beneficial depending on your gut bacteria composition, but there are cleaner sources of resistant starch. If you're not convinced to avoid beans yet, think about this—Pythagoras said, "*A fabis abstinete,*" meaning "Eat no beans."

DAIRY

All forms of dairy that contain protein (meaning everything except butter and ghee) cause problems for a substantial number of people, and most common industrial dairy products are outright Kryptonite for everyone. It's important to know that even if you eat Bulletproof forms of dairy, which we'll discuss next, if you consume sugar from milk in the morning you're not doing Bulletproof Intermittent Fasting. Only butter or ghee counts!

BULLETPROOF DAIRY
GRASS-FED, ORGANIC, RAW, FULL-FAT MILK, CREAM, OR YOGURT

Grass-fed raw milk gets mistreated by the media and by most health authorities, but this isn't warranted based on science. Properly treated raw dairy does not have significant microbiological problems. If it did, you probably wouldn't be here today, as your grandmother likely had raw dairy delivered every day in a glass bottle. Changes to the way animals are treated have caused the health risks. Today, conventional dairy cows are kept in unsanitary conditions. This is why illnesses from milk became such a large problem and the government began to require farms to pasteurize their milk in the first place. Because of the media smear, the first question most people ask about raw milk is "Is it safe?" The answer is that every food has some chance of making you sick, but raw milk is a lot less likely to do so than most other foods,

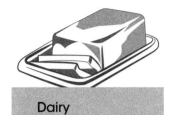

Dairy

BULLETPROOF

Bulletproof Ghee, organic grass-fed butter, colostrum

nonorganic grass-fed ghee or butter, organic grass-fed cream

organic grass-fed full-fat raw milk or yogurt

nonorganic grass-fed ghee or butter, organic grass-fed cream

grain-fed butter

skim or low-fat milk, fake butter, pasteurized nonorganic milk or yogurt

KRYPTONITE

all cheese, powdered milk, factory dairy, dairy replacer, condensed or evaporated milk, conventional ice cream

Dairy protein is a major source of allergies and inflamation. Test yourself to see what works. Ghee is safe for almost everyone, and butter usually is too because it is low in protein.

Download your free color copy at http://bulletproof.com/roadmap.

like chicken. The UK government has recently recommended that you not wash your chicken before cooking it because 75 percent of chicken has harmful bacteria on it that gets spread around your kitchen when you wash it. That is a lot more dangerous than anything found in raw milk! In a thorough examination of the research, Chris Kresser, an integrative health expert who has been interviewed on *Bulletproof Radio,* found that your risk of being hospitalized from drinking raw milk is 1 in 6 million.[21]

Raw milk is also nutritionally superior to regular milk, with more fat-soluble vitamins, minerals, and antioxidants. It also contains the enzyme lactase that helps people digest lactose, so it is more commonly tolerated than regular milk. You'll find beneficial bacteria in raw milk that can improve gut and mental function. As you read earlier, these bacteria are all killed during pasteurization, while pasteurization also modifies the proteins in milk so they become inflammatory. Homogenization is another process that damages the fat in the milk and removes an enzyme that helps with inflammation. Unhomogenized "cream top" milk is best. When a cow eats 100 percent grass instead of grains, the resulting milk has healthier fats, more nutrients, and fewer toxins.

In order to be considered Bulletproof, your dairy must therefore meet the following criteria:

1. Grass-fed and grass-finished, to increase the nutrient content and avoid antinutrients
2. Organic (where possible; most important is grass-fed), to avoid hormones, antibiotics, and pesticides
3. Raw, to preserve the nutrients, bacteria, and glutathione-boosting proteins (except butter, where raw matters less)
4. Full fat, because so many nutrients are in the fat and it is saturated fat

Because it is so difficult (and expensive) to find dairy products that meet these criteria and because many people still have digestive issues with dairy protein, I normally recommend avoiding all dairy except butter or ghee.

If you tolerate raw cream, you're lucky. Don't put it in your coffee, where it will be cooked. Whip it and use it for dessert, instead. Occasionally on my blog I link to sources of grass-fed dairy foods—like yogurt—that meet these criteria and you can order online: bulletproofexec.com/grassfeddairy.

KRYPTONITE DAIRY

PASTEURIZED, CONVENTIONAL, LOW-FAT, AND FAT-FREE DAIRY PRODUCTS

As you read earlier, pasteurization and homogenization destroy many of the nutrients and oxidize the fats in raw milk. Pasteurized milk competes only with gluten as the most allergic substance in the Western diet, and it's associated with a host of autoimmune conditions, osteoporosis, arthritis, heart disease, cancer, and autism. In many people, casein breaks down into casomorphin, which binds to the opiate receptors in your brain and causes food cravings and behavior changes. In the case of nonorganic pasteurized milk, you're also ingesting synthetic hormones, antibiotics, and possibly small amounts of GMO compounds from the grains fed to the cows.

In factory farms, the animals may be fed GMO grains, chicken beaks, sawdust, and sometimes even garbage and expired junk food, still in the wrapper. These cows are injected with antibiotics to increase milk production and keep them alive long enough to produce more milk and then be slaughtered. These antibiotics are transferred into the milk and into your body when you consume the dairy. If you care enough about your health and performance enough to pick up this book and read it, there's a clear case to stop supporting the way factory dairy mistreats animals and damages your health.

CHEESE

Cheese is the result of microbes such as bacteria or fungi competing for a food source. Each microbe attempts to use chemicals to convince other forms of life not to eat that food source. Sometimes we call those chemicals antibiotics or mold toxins; other times we call them "delicious." As your liver works to process cheese toxins, your Labrador brain demands energy, and you are likely to experience food cravings as a result. This is why so many people simply love cheese—they eat it, and then they crave more.

Mold toxins in cheese and dairy come from two places. The first is indirect contamination, which happens when dairy cows eat feed containing mycotoxins that pass into the milk. The more contaminated animal feed is, the cheaper it is, so producers don't normally strive to eliminate toxins from animal food. The second source of toxins in cheese comes from direct contamination, which occurs when we accidentally or intentionally introduce molds to cheese. The most common mycotoxins that are stable in cheese are citrinin, penitrem A, roquefortine C, sterigmatocystin, and aflatoxin. Some others, like patulin, penicillic acid, and PR toxin, are naturally eliminated from cheese. Sterigmatocystin is carcinogenic.[22] I'm not trying to be alarmist. Unless you have severe allergies, cheese is not going to kill you today. But it may cause inflammation in your skin and joints and brain, and it may make you fat. You choose whether or not to eat it.

POWDERED MILK

This stuff is made by spraying factory-farmed, pasteurized milk into a large heated chamber. The water in the milk evaporates, leaving a fine white powder made of protein, sugar, and a small amount of fat. Powdered milk has all the risks of regular pasteurized and factory-farmed dairy with the added problem of fat oxidation. In the United States, government subsidies have caused a huge stockpile of powdered milk to be produced, which is one reason the food industry keeps trying to sneak it into other foods.

CONDENSED MILK

Condensed milk is made by evaporating much of the water out of milk by heating it to high temperatures and then adding lots of sugar to make it sweet and thick. Preservatives, colorings, and other compounds are often added to prolong shelf life and make it appear more palatable. The cans that condensed milk is packaged in are also major sources of BPA and bromine. BPA is an estrogen mimetic, and bromine can block iodine absorption in the thyroid, leading to hypothyroidism.[23]

ICE CREAM

Unfortunately, ice cream has all the risks of regular factory-farmed dairy with the addition of high-fructose corn syrup, stabilizers, colorings, flavorings, preservatives, and all manner of non-Bulletproof ingredients. Even organic ice cream is high in sugar and milk proteins. But don't worry; you can make Bulletproof Creamy Coconut "Get Some" Ice Cream (page 282)!

PREPARED DAIRY PRODUCTS (AMERICAN CHEESE, COFFEE CREAMER, CHEESE SPREAD, CHEESE SAUCE, ETC.)

Coffee creamer is made with factory-farmed pasteurized dairy and is almost always served in a container lined with BPA and bromine. Cheese spreads (like Cheez Whiz) and cheese sauces are mostly cornstarch, sugar, orange colorings, and a host of other ingredients that are impossible to pronounce. Foods like these have nothing to offer in terms of nutrition and are filled with oxidized fats, toxins like MSG that induce brain fog, and possibly carcinogenic ingredients. #Notfood.

By now it should be pretty clear where you're going to spend most of your time on the Bulletproof Diet Roadmap—with vegetables, fats, and protein. If you stick to these categories most of the time, you'll get the greatest benefits. But if you avoid carbohydrates entirely, you're not going to like how you feel. The next chapter will steer you toward the most beneficial, Bulletproof sources of carbs so you can find the balance that works best for you

10

THE BULLETPROOF DIET ROADMAP TO SKETCHY NEIGHBORHOODS

The foods in this chapter—nuts, starches, and fruits—are ones you'll be eating in moderation on the Bulletproof Diet, but it's still incredibly important to choose wisely. These neighborhoods are sketchy, not outright dangerous. That means you want to visit them infrequently and use caution while you're there. Use this roadmap to find the versions of these foods that help you feel like your most powerful, awesome self instead of causing food cravings, brain fog, and weight gain even in small amounts.

These foods aren't unhealthy, but if you overeat them they're not going to help you reach your goals of eliminating food cravings, feeling awesome all the time, and looking great in your clothes. All of the foods here contain a significant amount of carbs and some antinutrients, so this is where timing really matters. When you're trying to lose weight, eating very few foods from these categories will be important, but when you're trying to maintain your weight, moderate amounts will work just fine. When I was working to lose weight, I ate almost no foods from these categories, but as I'm writing this book, I do eat a limited amount of Bulletproof starch several nights a week and one piece of fruit per day on occasion. If I wanted to lose weight tomorrow, I'd simply cut these out. This part of the diet is so predictable that it's almost programmable.

NUTS

Except for coconut, all nuts are Suspect to some extent, as they contain a high risk of mold contamination and toxins and high levels of omega-6 fats that oxidize easily and cause inflammation. If you're having trouble losing weight or suffering from headaches and joint pain while on the Bulletproof Diet, try removing nuts from your diet completely.

As you read earlier, nuts are high in antinutrients called phytates. To eliminate the phytates in your nuts, it's best to soak and/or sprout them. Most people (including me) don't have time to do this and do well on a handful of mold-free nuts. I recommend buying whole nuts with the skin (not shell) still on, as manufacturers use damaged

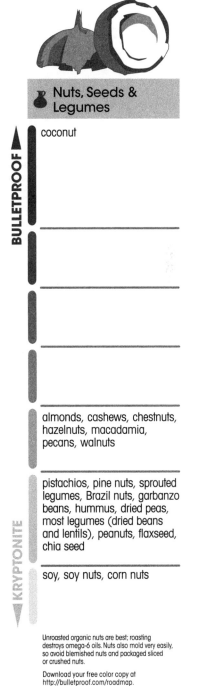

Nuts, Seeds & Legumes

BULLETPROOF

coconut

almonds, cashews, chestnuts, hazelnuts, macadamia, pecans, walnuts

pistachios, pine nuts, sprouted legumes, Brazil nuts, garbanzo beans, hummus, dried peas, most legumes (dried beans and lentils), peanuts, flaxseed, chia seed

soy, soy nuts, corn nuts

KRYPTONITE

Unroasted organic nuts are best; roasting destroys omega-6 oils. Nuts also mold very easily, so avoid blemished nuts and packaged sliced or crushed nuts.

Download your free color copy at http://bulletproof.com/roadmap.

nuts that are far more likely to contain mold toxins to make slivered, chopped, or ground nuts, nut butters, and nut flours. You'll get better oils if you buy refrigerated nuts, too, which are available in some health food stores. The nuts below are ranked according to their likelihood of mold, percentage of unsaturated fats, presence of antinutrients, and their total amount of carbohydrates.

BULLETPROOF NUTS

COCONUT

Coconut is one of the few sources of clean saturated fat and medium-chain fats from plants. These fats are anti-inflammatory, assist in fat-burning, and increase cognitive performance. Properly prepared, coconut is virtually free of antinutrients and is renowned for being antiallergenic. However, be careful when buying shredded coconut. In one study, about one-third of samples had a dangerous species of mold present.[1] When buying these products, go for high-end, unsweetened, larger flakes, which are less likely to have mold issues than smaller flakes. Whole coconuts, especially young Thai coconuts, are an amazing food with almost no carbs in the soft white meat, but coconut water is a major source of fructose. Save it for after dinner. Discard the meat and the water if the interior is gray or cloudy, as that is a sign of bacteria or mold having spoiled the coconut.

SUSPECT NUTS

RAW ALMONDS

Almonds are high in vitamin E, phytosterols, and antioxidants, but they're also relatively high in sugar, polyunsaturated oils, and phytates. Almonds are not going to satisfy you as well as you might expect.

CASHEWS

Mold is a definite issue with cashews because they're always boiled to remove the highly irritating outer layer of the nut. A study found 37 fungal species on Brazilian cashews, and the dominant species of mold was one that did form toxins.[2] Another study from Canada found 67 percent of cashews were contaminated with toxin forming molds.[3] Cashews are also fairly high in histamines. Choose fresh cashews sealed in a bag (not from a bin) and be wary of headaches, brain fog, food cravings, or joint pain after eating them.

HAZELNUTS

Hazelnuts are high in B vitamins, antioxidants, magnesium, potassium, and manganese. Eat them raw and in moderation so you don't consume too much polyunsaturated fat. Ninety percent of Egyptian hazelnuts tested in a study had aflatoxin, a cancer-causing, performance-sapping mold toxin, but the incidence in the United States or Europe is likely to be lower.[4]

MACADAMIA NUTS

These nuts are high in vitamin E, phosphorus, and potassium and should be totally Bulletproof, especially because there are almost no studies finding mold toxins on macadamias—but then again, there are almost no studies looking for them either. The major problem is that macadamias go rancid easily—buy them in the cold section if possible, and store them in the fridge. Macadamia oil has a high flash point, but it oxidizes easily, which is why I recommend not using it. Just eat the nuts when they're fresh!

PECANS

Pecans are high in thiamine, vitamin B$_6$, magnesium, manganese, phosphorus, and zinc, as well as antioxidants. The nuts absorb humidity from the air, which can cause mold to form, so buy them whole and store them sealed in

> I tried Bulletproof Coffee, and for the rest of that day I had through-the-roof energy, enthusiasm, and intuition. All this made for the natural high that I strive for now. I went from 250 pounds to now hovering around 170, and I'm entering my first 5-K. —**Kenneth**

the fridge or even freezer. Storage conditions really matter—I've had shelled pecans go bad in only 1 week of storage at room temperature at moderate humidity.

WALNUTS

Walnuts are very high in micronutrients but they are fairly high in histamines and have a higher risk of mold contamination than any other nut except Brazil nuts and pistachios.[5] Shelling your own walnuts helps a lot with this problem. Bonus points if you can crack a walnut with one of your biceps!

CHESTNUTS

Unlike most nuts, chestnuts are suspect because they're almost completely carbs, but they're high in B vitamins, vitamin C, and potassium and fairly low in antinutrients.

PINE NUTS

I grew up in New Mexico harvesting my own pine nuts, and they were amazing. Most of the pine nuts you can buy today come from China and are low quality and tend to have more mold problems. Studies show that mold toxins are present on various kinds on pine nuts, so I consider them all suspect.[6] I've mostly stopped eating them.

PISTACHIOS

To be fair, pistachios are high in several antioxidants and minerals, including B vitamins, magnesium, manganese, phosphorus, potassium, and zinc. However, pistachios are one of the nuts most commonly contaminated with

As an elite-level triathlete, I am constantly looking for an edge, and I am leaner and fitter than ever before, thanks to many small changes I have made through adopting the Bulletproof Diet. **—Adam O'Meara, professional athlete and Purica representative** mold toxins because the nuts open on the tree as they ripen, exposing them to aspergillus fungus. You have low odds of feeling great for hours with no food cravings after loading up on pistachios. That said, they're delicious.

BRAZIL NUTS

Brazil nuts are so high in linoleic acid that they're known for going rancid just a few days after being shelled, but the main problem with Brazil nuts is that they're one of the most mold-toxin-tainted nut products in existence. In fact, aflatoxin is so common in Brazil nuts that the European Union has set strict standards on the quantity and quality of Brazil nuts that are allowed into their countries.[7] Brazil nuts are high in selenium, but the amount varies greatly per nut, and it's not worth the toxin exposure to get the selenium.

KRYPTONITE NUTS

PEANUTS

Peanuts are actually a legume, but people often think they're a nut. The lectins in peanuts cause an inflammatory response in most people, with severe cases of allergies causing anaphylaxis and even death. These legumes are one of the most common carriers of aflatoxin,[8] and unlike most legumes, the lectins in peanuts are not destroyed by heat.[9] This means that the lectins are able to make their way into your bloodstream, where they cause inflammation and gut damage. Eating peanuts can increase intestinal mucus production by more than 40 percent—a level indicative of injury—and are also high in histamines. They have about the same amounts of nutrients as other legumes, but compared to animal products, they're nutritionally void. Peanuts also increase your level of very-long-chain saturated fats[10]—so long they don't fit in cell membranes—and this type of fatty acid is found more often in the brains of Alzheimer's sufferers.[11]

STARCHES

Starch is an energy store in food that is highly sought after in nature. There is usually a competition to get starch: Bugs want to eat it, bacteria want to eat it, and fungi want to eat it. That's not even to mention all the animals that want to eat it, too. For this reason, most plants have evolved complex defense systems to hold on to their starch. They are armor-plated with these antinutrients that make them harder for us to digest. But you do occasionally benefit from some starch, especially if you're on a heavy workout program. If you're sedentary or have a gut bacteria problem, you need less starch, but you still shouldn't avoid it entirely for long periods of time.

To put it simply: You'll lose weight if you avoid starch most of the time, but you won't feel great if you avoid starch all the time. It's also important to remember that you're not going to get much in the way of nutrients from most forms of starch. It's simply a source of fuel and basic building blocks. The answer is to eat limited amounts of the starches that are lowest in antinutrients. They appear below in order from the most nutritious with the least antinutrients and sugar to the ones that do far more harm than good.

BULLETPROOF STARCHES

PUMPKIN AND OTHER WINTER SQUASHES

Pumpkin is easily the most Bulletproof source of carbs because it's low in fructose and about as free of antinutrients as water. It's exceedingly high in potassium, carotenoids, and antioxidants, with moderate amounts of phosphorus, vitamin C, vitamin K, folate, zinc, magnesium, manganese, and calcium. Containing half a gram of soluble fiber, pumpkin will also nourish your gut bacteria without making you rush to the bathroom. Eat fresh pumpkin rather than canned. Canned pumpkin is often contaminated with BPA and is likely to contain other harmful ingredients as well.

SWEET POTATOES/YAMS

Sweet potatoes are a nutritious, tasty, low-toxin, and clean-burning starch. They're high in minerals, vitamins, and antioxidants, and have been a staple of traditional cultures for centuries. The fructose content of sweet potatoes is negligible, and compounds in sweet potato skin improve insulin sensitivity, HbA1C, cholesterol, and triglyceride levels in diabetic patients.[12]

CARROTS

Carrots are a good source of carot-enoids, potassium, calcium, phosphorus, vitamin C, vitamin K, antioxidants, and a little selenium. They're also high in polyacetylenes, which have been shown to inhibit cancer growth,[13] and anthocyanins, which improve brain function. Carrots are low in fructose and have no antinutrient content to speak of. However, they're very high in fiber. If you have irritable bowel syndrome or gut damage, opt for cooked carrots, which are easier to digest.

WHITE RICE

White rice is a grain, but it doesn't behave like other grains because it's quite low in antinutrients and is one of the lowest sugar starches. It is low in antinutrients because the outer layer that had the antinutrients has been removed. White rice is low in vitamins and minerals, so I mostly use it as a platform for butter, vegetables, sushi, and Brain Octane Oil; as fuel in the evening for sleep; and as a way of providing my gut bacteria with some food in the evening.

There is a real problem with arsenic contamination in white rice. To reduce your risk, buy high-quality brands and rinse the uncooked rice

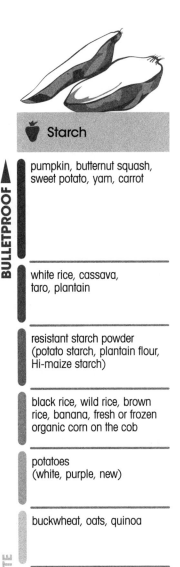

Starch

BULLETPROOF

pumpkin, butternut squash, sweet potato, yam, carrot

white rice, cassava, taro, plantain

resistant starch powder (potato starch, plantain flour, Hi-maize starch)

black rice, wild rice, brown rice, banana, fresh or frozen organic corn on the cob

potatoes (white, purple, new)

buckwheat, oats, quinoa

wheat, corn, millet, other grains, potato starch, corn starch, gluten-free powders

KRYPTONITE

Eat very few starchy foods—and it's most optimal in the evenings. Every 3 to 7 days, take one day to eat more. See the intake and eating times diagrams on page 89.

Download your free color copy at http://bulletproof.com/roadmap.

thoroughly. Gut bacteria will get some starch from any type of rice, but you can turn rice into their favorite food by cooking it and allowing it to cool, which forms resistant starch. You can also choose parboiled rice, which is better for your gut bacteria, or the most flavorful form of rice ever known, mochi. Mochi is steamed sticky white rice that's pounded into a hard square and cooled. You can buy it ready to bake in the refrigerator section at a natural foods grocery store, and they puff up into crunchy, chewy, hollow, amazing biscuitlike things that you can fill with butter or transform into a perfect waffle made of nothing but white rice! (These are not rice cakes.) Contrary to what most people expect, white rice is more Bulletproof than brown or wild rice, which I'll discuss in the Suspect section.

SUSPECT STARCHES

CASSAVA, TAPIOCA, AND TARO

These tropical woody shrubs are low in fructose but high in total carbs without much to offer nutritionally. They are also low in antinutrients, but when raw, they contain potentially deadly compounds. It's easy enough to prepare taro and cassava to remove these toxins, but if you're a raw foodist, watch out! It is possible to make a very-low-carb bread out of cassava, and it is a very healthy product. These are sources of resistant starch. Try taking them with a probiotic in the evening once you're in maintenance mode and see how you feel.

ORGANIC FRESH/FROZEN CORN ON THE COB

Corn is nearly universally contaminated, as it grows with a known toxin-forming mold called fusarium. When you get organic corn on the cob, the mold makes fewer toxins because herbicides like Roundup haven't been sprayed on the soil. Roundup causes agricultural molds to produce more toxins.[14] Corn is still a pretty-high-risk food, but it's better than most other grains as long as it's organic. Get it frozen, or when corn is in season, buy it from a farmer the same day it's picked.

BUCKWHEAT GROATS

These are technically a fruit. Some people find they tolerate buckwheat fine, while others react to it as badly. People with gut issues should heal themselves before experimenting with buckwheat, as the proteins in the hull can cross-react with other allergens.

OATS

Oats contain about the same amount of the antinutrient phytate as wheat, but fermenting oats seems to destroy much of it. Oats aren't heavily infected with agricultural molds, but studies show that organic oats have fewer mold toxins than conventional.[15] Oats also contain avenin, a prolamin protein similar to gluten that can cross-react with gluten and cause similar problems. For people with gut damage, all oats are Kryptonite. For everyone else, they're still not a good breakfast food!

BROWN, BLACK, AND WILD RICE

Many people believe wild rice is the best diet food around, but black and wild rice contain lots of antinutrients like phytate and lectins and gut-irritating fiber. We've all been told for years that eating more fiber is the key to digestive health, but certain types of fiber actually damage part of the lining of the gut called the intestinal villi. When intestinal villi get damaged, your ability to move nutrients through the digestive tract goes down. White rice tastes better than brown, black, and wild rice; doesn't cause the same digestive issues; and is lower in antinutrients. That said, wild rice tastes good. There isn't a good reason to choose brown rice over white.

QUINOA

Just like soy, this starch is all the rage in the vegetarian and vegan communities, for one good reason: It has no gluten. It's superior to most other grains, but it can still be irritating to the gut. It does have all of the amino acids you need for muscle growth, but in such small amounts that it would be difficult to eat enough quinoa to get the benefits. A serving of quinoa has 3 grams of protein while a serving of beef has 26 grams. Don't think of it as being a source of useful protein in your diet. It is a starchy grain, and quinoa suffers from the same limitations of all stored grains— they start to spoil in the field and then continue to do so once stored. Quinoa may not as bad as wheat, but it's not the be-all and end-all that some people want it to be.

POTATO STARCH

This resistant starch can boost healthy gut bacteria in some people when taken at night with a probiotic. It makes other people feel awful and causes brain fog and swelling. You can take advantage of this advanced biohack by experimenting with resistant starch only in the evening once you're in maintenance mode.

KRYPTONITE STARCHES

CONVENTIONALLY GROWN CORN

Corn is one of the most contaminated crops in terms of mold, thanks to GMOs and Roundup herbicide, which increases toxicity of naturally occurring field fungus. Corn also contains zein, a prolamin-rich protein that can cross-react with gluten and irritate people with gut issues. It's okay to have some organic, very fresh or frozen corn on the cob every once in a while, but corn bread, corn mash, polenta, and other processed dried corn products are Kryptonite.

WHEAT/GLUTEN-CONTAINING GRAINS

You've already read that wheat is bad for you because it spikes your blood sugar, hurts your gut, contains mold toxins, decreases your mental performance, and is addictive. Wheat starch causes a much larger spike in blood sugar than glucose or sucrose, resulting in massive blood sugar swings. The gluten and other proteins in wheat can damage your gut lining, depending on your genetics. Gluten is well known to contribute to a host of autoimmunity conditions where your body's immune system attacks itself, and some of those conditions, like Hashimoto's thyroiditis or lupus, can take years to form, so you won't feel it happening when you eat gluten. Wheat is also often contaminated with mold toxins that impact your performance and health in all the ways we've already discussed. The proteins in wheat are metabolized into gluteomorphins, which are an opioid. This is one of the reasons people find it so hard to give up bread. That craving you feel for bread is caused by the same mechanism that makes opiate addicts want more. Gluten also lowers cerebral blood flow, which is bad if you want your brain to work well.

MILLET

Millet is gluten-free, but it contains proteins that are similar to gluten and can cause gut damage and inflammation. Like most other grains that are stored for long periods of time, millet is often contaminated with mold toxins. Perhaps most harmful, millet causes thyroid damage more than any other food in people who are susceptible to it.[16] Millet contains goitrogens, substances that suppress the thyroid by interfering with iodine uptake. This can in turn create an enlargement of the thyroid or goiter. Sadly, grains just aren't very good foods for humans.

CORNSTARCH

Unlike nearly every other corn product except corn syrup, cornstarch is so heavily processed that it doesn't pose a major risk of mold toxins. However, it tends to have a negative impact on blood sugar and isn't a good source of food for gut bacteria. A major exception here is resistant cornstarch, which is

I've battled depression for years. Even though I've had a lot of success with therapy and supplements, I still experienced vicious mood swings. A few months after I went gluten-free and sugar-free on Bulletproof, I realized I wasn't having those huge crashes and crying fits. In fact, I wasn't having extreme mood swings at all. Being Bulletproof has given me the most mental clarity, stability, and focus I've probably had in my whole life. I'm a believer in the Bulletproof lifestyle, and so is my fiancée, who manages her rheumatoid arthritis without meds by staying away from grains and sugar. Thank you, Bulletproof Exec! —**Barry** cornstarch that is highly purified and modified so that it serves as food for bacteria in the gut. This is a highly refined type of corn. Even if it is made from GMO corn, there is no protein remaining, and I have lab tested resistant cornstarch and found it to be remarkably free of mold toxins. Supporting the GMO industry isn't ideal, but this is the only GMO corn product I'd use.

Resistant cornstarch isn't a good idea if you have yeast issues (starch feeds yeast) or if you have been exposed to toxic mold recently, because a zero-starch diet can help people with mold symptoms. If you're looking for resistant starch, make sure to buy cornstarch that is specifically processed to be resistant cornstarch, and only consume it in the evening. You can cook with it, but when I use it, I mix 2 tablespoons in water and take it before bed with probiotics. I did this every night for a month to get my gut flora used to it, and it improved my sleep quality slightly without causing any weight gain or health issues. Your mileage may vary with resistant starch, and it's not on the 14-day program.

FRUITS

Remember that, in general, fruits should be limited to the evenings because of their sugar content. The fruits below are ranked in order from the most nutritious fruits that are lowest in antinutrients and fructose to the ones with the highest fructose content, most common mold contamination, and fewest nutrients.

BULLETPROOF FRUITS

RASPBERRIES

Raspberries are low in sugar and one of the most micronutrient-dense fruits. They're very high in anthocyanins, polyphenols, and other antioxidants like ellagic acid, which can actually protect you from aflatoxin, the most dangerous cancer-causing mold toxin found in our food supply.[17] There are virtually no antinutrients in raspberries, though they tend to be a little higher in pesticides than some other fruits. However, even the most carefully picked and packed raspberries have a very short shelf life. Select firm, very fresh raspberries that are not at all mushy and avoid raspberries that are on sale, as grocery stores most often put them on sale when they're about to spoil but before you can see mold.

LEMONS AND LIMES

Lemons are low in toxins and contain antioxidants that can help your liver detox. For a Bulletproof drink, try squeezing lemons or limes into sparkling water.

CRANBERRIES

Although cranberries are usually made into dried fruit, juice, and other non-Bulletproof processed foods, whole cranberry fruits are a good choice if you cook them yourself. They're high in vitamins, low in sugar, generally low in antinutrients, and haven't (yet) been subjected to genetic modification.

BLACKBERRIES

Blackberries are low in antinutrients and have respectable macro- and micronutrient profiles. They have similar spoilage and freshness issues as raspberries do—don't eat the mushy ones!

STRAWBERRIES

Strawberries are high in vitamins and antioxidants, but the downsides to

Fruit

BULLETPROOF

avocado, blackberries, coconut, cranberries, lemon, lime, raspberries

blueberries, pineapple, strawberries, tangerine

grapefruit, pomegranate

apple, apricot, cherries, figs, honeydew, kiwifruit, lychee, nectarine, orange, peach, pears, plums

bananas, dates, grapes, guava, mango, melons, papaya, passion fruit, persimmon, plantain, watermelon

cantaloupe

KRYPTONITE

raisins, dried fruit, fruit leather, jam, jelly, canned fruit

Download your free color copy at
http://bulletproof.com/roadmap.

strawberries are that they tend to be fairly high in pesticides and histamines. Buy organic and pay attention to how you feel after eating them. They also spoil fast—cut out mushy spots quickly.

PINEAPPLE

Pineapples are extremely low in antinutrients, including pesticides, and high in vitamins and antioxidants. Save them for dessert because they're somewhat high in sugar. They're also higher in histamines than most other fruits.

TANGERINES

These are high in vitamins and various antioxidants, and tend to be low in antinutrients and molds.

BLUEBERRIES

Blueberries are an extremely high-nutrient fruit that is also high in antioxidants and polyphenols, which are believed to have anticancer and cardioprotective effects. They're usually high in pesticides, so organic varieties are a good choice, but wild blueberries are the best option. The polyphenols in blueberries, like the ones in coffee and chocolate, can help you to grow Bacteroidetes (thin-people bacteria). Also like coffee, blueberries increase a compound called brain-derived neurotrophic factor (BDNF) that is required in the brain for forming new connections. One problem with blueberries besides the pesticides is that it's hard to find frozen ones that aren't moldy. Companies sell the freshest blueberries right away and then freeze the older, moldy ones. If you don't feel well after eating frozen blueberries, it's probably because you ate mold toxins. Buy high-quality organic frozen or firm fresh blueberries. Frozen moldy berries are a much bigger problem than people realize.

SUSPECT FRUITS

POMEGRANATE

Fresh pomegranate juice has been shown to decrease LDL cholesterol oxidation, platelet aggregation, and other markers of atherosclerosis.[18]

Unfortunately, pomegranate juice and even the seeds are too high in sugar to be consumed in large amounts.

GRAPEFRUIT

Grapefruit contains spermidine and polyamine, which can cause headaches and allergic-like reactions in susceptible people. However, spermidine may be beneficial for those who can tolerate it, as some animal studies indicate it may prevent some effects of aging.[19] Grapefruit is low in antinutrients overall, but it contains a compound called naringin, which can interfere with the way your liver detoxes substances like medications and petrochemicals. This is why your medications may carry warnings to forgo grapefruit. Depending on the health of your liver and your stress levels, grapefruit may not be a great idea. I don't intentionally slow down my detox pathways!

HONEYDEW AND WATERMELON

These melons are high in vitamins and antioxidants and low in antinutrients and pesticides. Enjoy a moderate-sized piece of these very-fast-digesting sugar bombs for dessert after dinner only, but wait a little while because you don't want them in your stomach at the same time as protein and fat since they digest so quickly. If they move into the lower intestine with other foods and ferment, it can cause digestive distress. You can eat them on an empty stomach in moderation, but you will still experience a big burst of blood sugar.

APPLES

Some people are allergic to certain proteins in apples, so it's important to see how you feel when adding apples back into your diet after the first 2 weeks. Apples are high in several antioxidants that are believed to help protect against cancer and heart disease, but the biggest problem with apples is their pesticide content. Apples are ranked number 1 on the Environmental Working Group's 2014 list of 12 most-contaminated fruits and vegetables. You should try to buy organic apples whenever possible, and wash any nonorganic ones thoroughly before consumption.

APRICOTS

These are an excellent source of carotenoids, antioxidants, and micronutrients, with a fairly low antinutrient load. Unfortunately, they're often contaminated with pesticides. For this reason, you should buy organic apricots whenever possible and thoroughly wash the nonorganic varieties. It's also a good idea to remove the skin. Eat them for dessert—they're full of fructose.

CHERRIES

These fruits have high nutrient content and a high glucose load. They're also usually contaminated with a fair amount of pesticides. There are several studies showing tart cherry juice reduces inflammation, cholesterol, and triglycerides and reduces body-fat accumulation when fed to rats,[20,21] but cherries themselves do have a lot of sugar and should be eaten in moderation.

KIWIFRUIT

Kiwifruit is high in nutrients, but has more fructose and histamines than many other fruits. The seeds of kiwifruit also act as a mild blood thinner and may protect against blood clots.

NECTARINES

Nectarines taste amazing, but they are mostly bags of sugary water that are high in fructose. They're also higher in pesticides than most fruits. To reduce the pesticide risk, buy organic nectarines or wash conventional ones very well.

ORANGES

Oranges are very high in sugar. In fact, with 50 percent more fructose than nectarines, oranges are truly watery candy. Plus, the antioxidants in oranges tend to degrade after they're picked. One good thing about oranges is that they have almost no antinutrients and an average pesticide load since the rind blocks a good deal of the pesticides from reaching the fruit.

PEACHES

Peaches should be left at room temperature or they become less sweet, but make sure to eat them before they mold. Ranking at number 5 on the EWG's 2014 list of most contaminated foods, peaches are high in pesticides. The fuzz on peach skin traps the pesticides and the skin is soft, allowing the pesticides to be absorbed into the fruit. Buy organic whenever you can.

PEARS

Pears are one of the most hypoallergenic foods on the planet, so almost everyone can tolerate them. Pears have a moderate amount of pesticide contamination and are higher in fructose than many other fruits, so they should be eaten in small amounts.

PLUMS

Plums are high in nutrients and fiber and contain sorbitol, which can help with constipation. They have almost no endogenous antinutrients, but they're often sprayed with pesticides. Luckily, they're only 17th out of 51 tested plants for pesticides, according to the EWG.

FIGS

Figs are extremely high in sugar, but they do have some health benefits, including polyphenols and even calcium. They are low in antinutrients, but they do rot easily if left out. Freshness really matters for figs. Unfortunately, figs are too high in fructose to eat on a regular basis.

LYCHEES

Lychees are high in nutrients and antioxidants, but their antioxidant levels decline with storage and/or browning. They're also high in sugar and should be eaten in moderation.

PASSION FRUIT

Passion fruit is suspect because it's higher in calories and carbs than most other fruits. The good news is that it's relatively low in fructose. Passion fruit is high in iron, potassium, phosphorus, folate, and carotenoids and has a decent amount of soluble fiber.

PAPAYA

Papaya is high in some nutrients and fairly low in pesticides, but it's often genetically modified. My blood tests show that I'm actually allergic to papaya, which is odd considering I don't really like it and have only eaten papaya maybe 20 times in my life. Normally, allergies develop after more frequent repeated exposures. There's no test or study that shows this, but I believe that my allergy to papaya may have developed because it's so commonly genetically modified. See how you feel after eating papaya. I avoid it entirely.

PLANTAINS

Since they're so high in calories, carbs, and sugar, these should be thought of more as a starch than a fruit. Their high fructose load precludes them from being a staple, but plantains are useful as a form of resistant starch, only to be eaten at night with probiotics.

BANANAS

Everyone's favorite fruit—the banana—is about as nutrient dense as white potatoes with a similar nutritional profile. They are high in carbs and low in most nutrients. Despite their convenience, bananas are too high in fructose and carbs to be Bulletproof and should be eaten after dinner only every now and then.

FRESH DATES

Dates are high in calcium, potassium, magnesium, and carotenoids, but they're extremely high in fructose. Dried dates are a common source of mold. There isn't any great benefit to be had from dates, so it's best to eat other foods that are more Bulletproof.

GRAPES

Grapes are another high-fructose, low-benefit fruit. The supposed benefits of resveratrol and other antiaging substances in grapes are mostly overblown extrapolations from the French "paradox" (the idea that the French suffer low rates of heart disease because they drink lots of wine— it's probably because they eat lots of butter!). Grapes and raisins in particular are sources of the mold toxin aflatoxin.

GUAVA

Guava is very high in soluble fiber, which can help with constipation if that's a problem for you. Pink guava also have twice the amount of lycopene as tomatoes. This is another fruit that's unfortunately too high in sugar to be Bulletproof.

MANGO

Mango is high in calcium, phosphorus, potassium, vitamin C, fiber, folate, beta-carotene, and more than 25 different carotenoids, some of which have been shown to inhibit cancer formation in vitro. It's also delicious, but very high in sugar, so eat in moderation. Mango has an extremely high glycemic index. When I was fat, I noticed that I got really angry and moody after eating mango because my blood sugar was spiking and crashing so drastically. Now that I'm Bulletproof I can eat mango once in a while, but if I were in weight-loss mode I would cut it out entirely.

CANTALOUPE

Cantaloupes are extremely high in sugar and are one of the moldiest fruits in the world, so unless you've got a freshly cut, perfectly ripe, unblemished one, it's worth skipping. The moldy nature of cantaloupes has proven useful in the past, however. When scientists were first developing penicillin as a vaccine, they conducted a search and found that a strain of penicillin from a moldy cantaloupe in a Peoria market produced the largest amount of penicillin when grown in the deep vat in submerged conditions.

PERSIMMON

These are high in calcium, phosphorus, potassium, and vitamin C, and tend to be fairly low in toxins, mold, and pesticides, but they are too high in sugar to eat every day. Persimmons are very high in a polyphenol called tannic acid, which is used to tan leather. Some tannic acids, such as grape-seed extract, are good for you, but an excess of tannic acids can cause digestive distress and a numb tongue.

KRYPTONITE FRUITS

RAISINS, FRUIT LEATHER, AND OTHER DRIED FRUITS

Dried fruit is higher in calories, carbs, sugar, and fructose than regular fruit, plus it's often depleted of fruit's beneficial compounds. Dried fruit is also often treated with preservatives like sodium benzoate and colorings like Red #40 to make them look more appealing. Even worse, dried fruit is well known to have higher levels of mold toxins as a result of the drying process, which means that you'll experience a double dose of food cravings as your liver works to detox the mold and the fructose at the same time.

CANNED FRUIT

Canned fruit is no better than canned vegetables. It's often treated with colorings and preservatives to make it look fresh and is often suspended in thick fructose syrup. The fruit used for canning is often lower quality or blemished, which means it's more likely to contain some moldy fruit. Many of the nutrients are also lost during conventional canning, when the fruit is subjected to high pressure and heat. The cans themselves present another problem, as the syrup dissolves and absorbs things like bromine and BPA that block iodine absorption and interfere with hormone levels.

There is no benefit from canned fruit over regular fruit, and the high sugar and toxin content make it Kryptonite.

JAMS, JELLIES, AND PRESERVES

These are cooked at high temperatures under high pressure, which destroys most of the beneficial antioxidants and nutrients in the fruit. After processing, what's left is almost pure sugar, and most fruit preserves have tons of added sweeteners, stabilizers, and preservatives. To top it all off, the fruit that's used to make preserves is usually the "cast off" fruit that couldn't be sold in stores because it was starting to go bad. It's possible to make your own jam using fresh fruits and organic sugar, and I noticed a substantial difference in how I felt after eating jams made from high-quality ingredients. But even homemade preserves naturally contain a huge amount of sugar. You can probably get away with having some on a protein fasting day if you're not dealing with a major health issue, but you shouldn't eat them all the time.

Unfortunately, nuts, starches, and fruits are not the staples of a healthy diet. With a few exceptions such as white rice, starchy vegetables, and resistant starch, most starch is basically sugar that feeds yeast in the body. It needs to be timed and portioned carefully. Nuts are delicious and convenient, but freshness, unstable fats, and antinutrients are all major issues. For much of the time I spent working to become Bulletproof, I ate large amounts of nuts, but I found that my health and performance increased when I eliminated them. Now I eat them as an occasional treat. Speaking of treats, carbs and fruits should be seen as desserts instead of a major source of nutrition. Eating fruit at the height of summer is an amazing experience, and now that I'm happy with my weight I'll eat well over 25 grams of fructose at a strawberry festival without feeling the slightest bit guilty, but it's important to keep in mind that fruits are unrelated to vegetables and more like candy. Especially during the 2-week Bulletproof program, it's important to avoid fruits as much as possible.

THE BULLETPROOF DIET ROADMAP TO RED-LIGHT NEIGHBORHOODS

The categories in this chapter—spices and flavorings, sweeteners, and beverages—are the places on the Bulletproof Diet roadmap that will add flavor and excitement to your diet. They are necessary for enjoyment and the art of food, but eating too much of them or the wrong ones can make you feel sluggish, weak, and bloated—basically as if you had a bad hangover! Most people don't think about which flavorings they use or what they drink when considering their diet or performance, but the truth is that many common drinks contain harmful ingredients that are making you tired, fat, and desperate for more sugar, while even the dried spices you use at home can play a major role in the way you look, feel, and perform.

When I started working really hard on being healthy, I switched from regular soda to diet soda. One hot day as I was rushing off to class, I stopped and got a 32-ounce diet soda. I drank the whole thing before the lecture started, and as I was sitting in class, I started feeling extremely light-headed and drugged, to the point that I actually drooled on myself a little bit. I was addled. The only thing I had done differently that day was drink such a large diet soda, and this made me start paying attention to what diet soda did to me. When I cut it out of my diet, I felt a tremendous decrease in food cravings. I realized it was because I'd stopped allowing the chemicals in the soda to throw my Labrador brain into a panic. Drinking that huge dose of diet soda allowed me to feel what it was actually doing to me all the time.

In my research I found that many flavorings, sweeteners, and beverages were actually doing the same thing to my brain as the diet soda. I experimented with eliminating different spices from my diet to determine which ones helped me think, feel, and look better and which caused food cravings and brain fog. They're all arranged here in order from the most beneficial to the most harmful. Let's take a look at some of the best and worst sources of flavor, sweetness, and hydration.

SPICES AND FLAVORINGS

Most herbs and spices have health benefits and antioxidant function. It's also common for them to have a healthy impact on your gut flora. But many common spices and herbs have psychoactive compounds that were originally used for medicinal purposes. The arrangement of herbs and spices and other flavorings here is designed to maximize the health benefits of spices, minimize antinutrient exposure, and keep you firmly in charge of your own biology.

The herb and spice industry is painfully aware of spoilage issues, which is why it's become so common to irradiate spices. This process exposes them to radiation so they become sterilized. Irradiation destroys many of the antioxidant and health benefits of herbs and spices, and irradiated or not, herbs and spices can spoil easily in your own home. Herbs often contain naturally strong antifungal and antibacterial oils, so the species that can flourish on them are usually the most aggressive toxins. When you get that canister of paprika down from the back shelf, pry it open, and dump some into a steaming pot of food, you're likely putting a substantial amount of toxin in, too. You'll always find a few mold spores in natural products, and the environment in your spice cabinet above the stove is a perfect incubator. One of the simplest things you can do to increase your performance is to toss out spices that more than a few months old. Use high-quality, recently opened, fresh or dried herbs and spices, or don't use them at all. I've done my best to identify the rationale behind the rankings in this section, but there is always room for personal experimentation. It's up to you to decide where you go on the roadmap and how that makes you feel and perform.

BULLETPROOF SPICES AND FLAVORINGS

APPLE CIDER VINEGAR

One study found that 20 grams of apple cider vinegar reduces glucose levels and insulin sensitivity after a meal in both insulin resistant and healthy people.[1] There's also evidence that it can improve cardiovascular function, fight tumors, and kill pathogens.[2] This is the only vinegar I use in my kitchen besides white distilled vinegar.

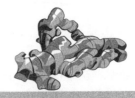

Spices & Flavorings

BULLETPROOF ▲

Bulletproof Chocolate Powder, ground vanilla extract, apple cider vinegar, cilantro, coffee*, ginger*, parsley, sea salt

lavender, oregano, rosemary, thyme, turmeric

all-spice, cinnamon, cloves,* organic prepared mustard with no additives

mustard seed, onion, table salt

black pepper,* conventional chocolate, garlic,* nutmeg,* paprika*

miso, tamari, tofu

KRYPTONITE ▼

commercial dressings, spice mixes and extracts, MSG, yeast, caseinate, textured protein, bouillon and broth, hydrolyzed gluten, anything labeled enzyme modified flavoring or seasoning

* Beware, these items often harbor toxic mold species. It's best to use fresh, high-quality options whenever you can.

Download your free color copy at http://bulletproof.com/roadmap.

SEA SALT

As you learned in the myths section in Chapter 2, in the right form salt presents a number of benefits and can help you manage stress. I regularly consume 5 to 8 grams of sea salt a day.

FRESH GINGER

Ginger is a potent anti-inflammatory that's been used for centuries as a way to reduce fevers as well as swelling from cuts and bruises. Watch out for the powdered ginger you're likely to find at the store, especially in the bulk bins, as it's often exposed to excessive humidity and spoilage. Potent immune-system suppressants have been discovered in ginger molds.[3]

OREGANO

This herb is high in antioxidants and plant phenolics, and has some medicinal benefits when it comes to helping the gut biome and suppressing yeast in your body. As long as you buy from high-quality sources and don't shake the container over steam (which traps water and allows mold to grow on any spice), oregano is an amazing herb. I use it as a crust on meat instead of black pepper.

TURMERIC

Turmeric provides one of the most potent anti-inflammatories you can get from food. It's extremely high in carotenoids, which is what gives it a yellow hue, and has been used for centuries to help heal wounds, fight infections, and even decrease the risk of cancer. There is still ongoing research into the positive effects of turmeric, but it's well documented to help your gut biome, reduce inflammation, and thin the blood. Turmeric can even protect your body from the mold toxin aflatoxin![4]

ROSEMARY

Carnosic acid, the active ingredient in rosemary, has been shown to protect brain cells from inflammation in vitro,[5] and some people believe that rosemary boosts brain function. Rosmarinic acid, another major active ingredient in rosemary, has protective effects on your glucose and lipid metabolism.[6] Another study indicated that rosemary helps combat rheumatoid arthritis.[7] Rosemary is exceptionally low in toxins and prevents fat oxidation. In a marinade, rosemary will protect unstable oils in meat, while using it in sautés will keep delicate oils intact for longer.[8]

THYME

Thyme has antifungal and antioxidant effects, and works almost as well as rosemary to protect delicate fats in your food from oxidation during cooking.[9]

ORGANIC PREPARED MUSTARD WITH NO ADDITIVES

The prepared mustards you're likely to find at most restaurants are loaded with fillers, artificial colorings, corn syrup, MSG, and often vegetable oils and other ingredients that decrease your performance. Try to find high-quality organic mustard with no additives or sugar.

VANILLA

More than just a popular scent for air fresheners, real vanilla can actually boost your brainpower! Vanilla contains chemicals called vanilloids that activate receptors, reduce inflammation, and improve mental performance. For centuries, it has been used to calm stomach pains, reduce hunger pangs, and relieve stress. Europeans believed in vanilla's abilities to reduce joint pain and help digestion. Pregnant South Pacific Island women used vanilla to reduce the nausea of morning sickness. More recent research has claimed that vanilla can increase penile blood flow, at least in older men.[10] Vanilla also has one of the highest ORAC (oxygen radical absorbance capacity) scores, which measure a food's antioxidant content.[11]

The problem is that the anti-inflammatory compounds in vanilla are destroyed by excess heat. If the vanilla pods or powder are improperly

> This morning I added ½ teaspoon of vanilla to my Bulletproof Coffee mixed directly in with the brewed coffee, not in with the coffee grounds. I feel like a blanket that I didn't even know was there has been pulled off of my brain. If the butter and Brain Octane Oil were a lubricant and restorative, then adding the vanilla could be described as a clarifier/ electrifier. —**Seth**

processed and/or exposed to higher than optimal temperatures, the benefits are lost, and heating vanilla poses another problem, mold toxins. The compounds in vanilla that help improve cognitive performance also act as natural antifungal agents. When these compounds are destroyed, mold spores and fungi are able to grow on the dried beans during storage. Vanilla is a powerful flavoring agent for your food and your brain, but if you eat the wrong kind of vanilla, it can actually cause more harm than good.[12]

Most people have rarely if ever had real vanilla powder; instead they get synthetic vanillin.

CHOCOLATE

Typical chocolate bars are Kryptonite because of their added sugar, milk products, and artificial flavorings, but very dark chocolate itself is actually quite healthy. Chocolate is full of polyphenols and antioxidants that fight free radicals and has a mild amount of caffeine to enhance performance. Research shows that 85 percent dark chocolate raises healthy HDL cholesterol levels without affecting insulin resistance, inflammation, or weight gain.[13] But there are risks. All chocolate is produced by fermentation, and 80 percent of South American chocolate sampled had mold contamination.[14] Sixty-four percent of the microbes that ferment chocolate create mold toxins.[15] European chocolate tends to be lowest in mold toxins, as they have stricter limits. Choose your chocolate wisely, make sure it's at least 85 percent dark chocolate, and enjoy! I almost always take coconut charcoal with chocolate to bind some of the mold toxins—mold in chocolate is at least as common as it is in coffee.[16]

SUSPECT SPICES AND FLAVORINGS

BLACK PEPPER

Despite being one of the most common spices, studies have shown that black pepper tends to be especially high in mold toxins,[17] particularly aflatoxin and ochratoxin A.[18] I love the taste of it, but I noticed that when I ate a lot of black pepper I woke up with sore joints, which for me is a sign of mold exposure. Since the risk is so high, I generally recommend avoiding it. If you continue to eat black pepper, ditch the ground stuff, as it is far moldier and the essential oils are gone. A good pepper grinder with fresh, high-end black pepper is the only way to do it. I've switched to oregano mostly.

NUTMEG

A significant percentage of nutmeg is high in mold toxins, but we don't need to pay attention to that because the toxic dose of nutmeg *itself* is only 2 teaspoons.[19] It has its own onboard toxins, and you'll feel them at even $\frac{1}{2}$ teaspoon. Small amounts are unlikely to cause big problems, but it's best to look for high-quality brands and use it sparingly. I've experienced noticeable stuttering from consuming $\frac{1}{2}$ teaspoon of nutmeg in eggnog.

TABLE SALT (PURE SODIUM CHLORIDE)

Regular table salt has been refined to remove all of the nutrients, but the real problem with table salt is its fillers and anticaking agents. To be sure you aren't ingesting any unwanted chemicals and are getting trace minerals, use sea salt, instead.

ALL OTHER VINEGARS (EXCEPT APPLE CIDER VINEGAR)

While flavorful, most vinegars contain significant amounts of yeast and fungal by-products that function as antinutrients and can limit your performance. Red wine vinegar, malt vinegar, and balsamic vinegar tend to be highest in antinutrients, including mold toxins and in the case of balsamic, lead. I was astounded to feel a difference when I switched from large amounts of balsamic vinegar to apple cider vinegar in salad dressing.

KRYPTONITE SPICES AND FLAVORINGS

FERMENTED SOY, TAMARI, AND MISO

As you already know, in almost every form except lecithin and natto (which undergo bacterial fermentation), soy has a host of problems. Even in small amounts, these foods act as Kryptonite, providing histamines and causing inflammation, allergies, thyroid problems, osteoporosis, hormone problems, and poor brain function. #Notfood.

COMMERCIAL SALAD DRESSINGS

These are carefully crafted symphonies of engineered food cravings, usually made with refined oils, artificial flavors, spices, unlabeled MSG, and cheap preservatives. Low-fat versions often have artificial sweeteners like aspartame, too.

YEASTS

Some vegans use nutritional yeast and other yeast products as dairy replacements. By definition, yeasts—which are fungi—almost always contain high levels of toxins. When you eat yeast, it encourages candida to grow in your body and changes the fungal biome of your gut. The toxin production of yeasts is so great that even the FDA has acknowledged the problem.[20] When you eat toxins from yeast, or even worse, when yeast in your gut generates toxins, you'll experience food cravings and energy lags. There is also an association between baker's and brewer's yeast and heart disease. If you want to be Bulletproof, it's best to avoid all yeasts.

MSG

Of all the food additives, flavorings, and preservatives in modern food, MSG might be the worst in terms of its effects on cognitive performance. Years ago, the food industry managed to sneak in a ruling that any substance less than 75 percent MSG by weight does not need to be labeled as MSG. In response, chemical companies now make "spices" that are 74 percent MSG by weight that can be used with impunity in foods that are labeled "no added

MSG." These companies also make sure that the MSG forms as the result of glutamate combining with sodium, rather than adding MSG itself, as it would then need to be identified. Sneaky! Check out the Bulletproof Web site bulletproofexec.com/MSG for a list of hidden sources of MSG.

ARTIFICIAL FLAVORS

Artificial flavors are often produced from petrochemicals and often have unpredictable (but never helpful) effects on your liver and brain. Most are not adequately tested, and they are often found in foods that also contain high-fructose corn syrup, MSG, and other toxins. They have been linked to ADHD and behavioral issues in children and can cause cognitive problems in adults as well.

SWEETENERS AND SUGARS

Sweeteners are controversial in most diets, as there is some evidence that even a sweet taste in your mouth that you don't swallow could have an effect on your insulin. However, sweet flavors are a part of some recipes and provide a complete food experience. After extensive research I settled on the list of Bulletproof sweeteners below, and have been using some of them reliably for a decade. See how they work for you.

BULLETPROOF SWEETENERS AND SUGARS

XYLITOL FROM NORTH AMERICAN HARDWOOD

This sugar alcohol, which you can purchase as an extract, is found in many fruits and vegetables and is well tolerated by almost everyone. It's sweeter than table sugar but has a negligible effect on your insulin. If you eat too much xylitol before your body is used to digesting it or eat GMO corn–based xylitol from China, you might experience "disaster pants" or its little cousin "tornado flatulence." If you eat a little bit of xylitol on a regular basis, your body will digest it with no problem. Women who use xylitol have less osteoporosis, and xylitol is well known to inhibit cavities, tooth decay, and even sinus infections.[21] I've been using it to make ice cream for years, and

I squirt a xylitol solution in my sinuses before I fly to keep the risk of bacterial sinus problems down. The argument against xylitol is that it *may* have negative effects on your gut flora, but I believe the benefits outweigh the risks. It's also delicious in Bulletproof Coffee!

ERYTHRITOL

This is another natural sugar alcohol found in fruits and vegetables. It's about 60 to 70 percent as sweet as regular sugar but has zero calories and carbs and no effect on glucose or insulin levels. Erythritol is far less likely to cause gastric discomfort than other sugar alcohols. As with xylitol, it's best to find a non-GMO version. I often mix erythritol and xylitol 50/50 to get a smoother flavor.

STEVIA

This plant is growing in popularity as a sugar substitute and has been used in Japan for decades. Farmers used to pick the leaves off the stevia plant and chew them like gum. The extract of stevia has a bittersweet flavor, which some people love and others dislike. Stevia is considered safe as a sweetener and has been shown to improve blood glucose control and help diabetic patients manage their blood sugar levels.

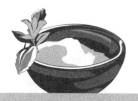

Sweeteners

BULLETPROOF ▲

xylitol, erythritol, stevia

sorbitol, maltitol, and other sugar alcohols

non-GMO dextrose, glucose, raw honey

maple syrup, coconut sugar

white sugar, brown sugar, agave, cooked honey

fructose, fruit juice concentrate, high-fructose corn syrup

aspartame (NutraSweet), sucralose (Splenda), acesulfame potassium

▼ KRYPTONITE

Download your free color copy at http://bulletproof.com/roadmap.

SORBITOL, MALTITOL, AND OTHER SUGAR ALCOHOLS

These sweet compounds are usually sourced from plants. They do have laxative effects if overconsumed and a small effect on blood sugar level, but are still much better than regular table sugar.

NON-GMO DEXTROSE AND GLUCOSE

Glucose is the main type of sugar used by your body and a major source of energy for your brain. In fact, when you're not in ketosis, your brain runs almost entirely on glucose. Dextrose is a slightly larger molecule of glucose. Dextrose and glucose are absorbed easily into your bloodstream, which is why they're often used for testing for blood sugar control. Consuming too much of them is not a good idea, but small amounts can be useful for supporting brain function before a test, presentation, or a sporting event. Glucose and dextrose also contain zero fructose, which will keep your liver, gut, and brain happy. Dextrose is used extensively in fermentation, so if you have yeast issues it will make you quite flatulent and should be avoided.

RAW HONEY

Raw honey contains antioxidants, enzymes, and nutrients, but cooking honey destroys many of these substances and transforms honey into something roughly akin to corn syrup. Raw honey can also be used as an antimicrobial, while cooked honey doesn't have the same effect. The main reason raw honey is on the Bulletproof Diet is because, as you read in Chapter 5, up to 1 tablespoon taken before bedtime can have a profoundly positive effect on sleep. Just a reminder, when you put raw honey in hot coffee, it isn't raw anymore! If you like your coffee sweet, use stevia or xylitol.

SUSPECT SWEETENERS AND SUGARS

MAPLE SYRUP

Pure maple syrup (not the fake stuff that's made of mostly high-fructose corn syrup) is a fairly low-fructose sweetener that's fine to eat on special occasions, like when you make gluten-free pancakes, but it shouldn't be used every day.

COCONUT SUGAR

Coconut sugar is almost all sucrose, with small amounts of fructose and glucose. It raises blood sugar less than regular table sugar and is very high in nutrients like iron, B vitamins, potassium, zinc, and magnesium. It's still sugar, though, so exercise caution when eating it.

WHITE SUGAR

Table sugar (sucrose) is a mix of equal parts glucose and fructose. When eaten in small amounts in the evening it won't cause much harm, but eating too much sucrose contributes to tooth decay, heart disease, diabetes, and obesity and feeds yeast in the body. The average American eats more than 70 pounds of sugar per year, which is obviously way too much. Avoiding sucrose is a great step toward becoming Bulletproof.

BROWN SUGAR

This is just like regular table sugar except it also has a small amount of added molasses, a by-product of sugar manufacturing. This produces more advanced glycation end products that accelerate aging and contribute to heart disease. This can decrease your performance on a day-to-day basis, so brown sugar should only be used on special occasions at night.

AGAVE SYRUP OR AGAVE NECTAR

Despite what you may have read on some health sites, agave syrup is not healthier than regular sugar. It's actually worse. Agave syrup or nectar is 70 to 90 percent fructose. In some ways, agave is even worse than sucrose-sweetened soda because it contains almost twice as much performance-robbing fructose.

KRYPTONITE SWEETENERS AND SUGARS

FRUCTOSE

One of the most important things to minimize on the Bulletproof Diet, fructose causes liver damage, toxin accumulation, advanced glycation end product formation, and fatty liver disease; contributes to obesity, intestinal overgrowth, gout, and fungal infections; and decreases brain function. Can you say "Kryptonite"?

FRUIT JUICE CONCENTRATE

There's nothing in fruit juice concentrate that you can't get from other foods, and it mainly serves as a major source of unwanted fructose. The lowest-quality, most moldy fruit is often used, resulting in the presence of aflatoxins, ochratoxin A, patulin, and *Alternaria* species.[22]

HIGH-FRUCTOSE CORN SYRUP

High-fructose corn syrup is made by refining GMO corn sugar into concentrated syrup and is then added to almost every food in the standard American diet. Health experts Dr. Robert Lustig and Gary Taubes, among others, have shown that HFCS is a major contributor to obesity, diabetes, hypertension, and gout. It damages your liver, decreases your mental performance, contributes to fungal infections, and makes you fat if consumed in anything but very small amounts. It is a major cause of food cravings.

ASPARTAME

As you read in Chapter 3, this artificial sweetener has been linked to numerous forms of cancer[23] (although this debate is still raging) and metabolizes into formaldehyde in your body, which is a known carcinogen. There is no good reason to introduce it to the high-performance machine that is your body! It is one of the top creators of food cravings.[24]

SUCRALOSE

Marketed as Splenda, this artificial sweetener is more similar to a pesticide than it is to sugar. Sucralose is made by substituting chlorine for some of the molecules in regular sugar, creating a molecule structurally related to polychlorinated biphenyls (PCBs), a known carcinogen. About 15 percent of the sucralose you ingest is stored in your body, and no one knows what it does or where it goes after that. There haven't been any long-term safety studies on sucralose, and there is some animal evidence suggesting it may be harmful. It wreaks havoc on healthy gut bacteria, too.[25]

ACESULFAME POTASSIUM (ACE-K)

This artificial sweetener is found in Diet Coke, among other products. There have been very few studies on the safety of ace-K in humans, and researchers are concerned about it.[26] This is scary, and my personal experiences with ace-K are even scarier. I developed benign nodules on my thyroid from consuming high amounts of ace-K in the late '90s when on an Atkins-style diet. This is a commonly reported side effect, and my nodules went away when I quit using ace-K.

BEVERAGES

I'm very sorry to tell you this, but there is no such thing as Bulletproof alcohol. While some types of alcohol are better than others, they all absolutely give you food cravings, brain fog, and reduced resilience. I don't like it, but it's what the research shows and what my clients report after giving up alcohol for a month. For your first 2 weeks on the Bulletproof Diet, try not to drink alcohol at all so you can see how your brain

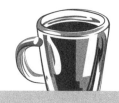

💭 Beverages

BULLETPROOF ▲

Coffee made from Bulletproof Coffee beans, high quality green tea, diluted coconut milk, mineral water in glass

---

filtered water with lime/lemon, green tea

---

tap water with lime/lemon, water with muddled fruit, fresh brewed iced tea – unsweetened, fresh nut milk

---

kombucha, raw milk, bottled iced tea–no sugar added, fresh coconut water, coconut water (bottle/box), bottled nut milks

---

freshly squeezed fruit juice

---

pasteurized milk

KRYPTONITE ▼

soy milk, packaged juice, diet drinks, soda, sweetened drinks, aspartame drinks, sports drinks

Download your free color copy at http://bulletproof.com/roadmap.

performs. Once you're in maintenance mode, you can drink from the list of Suspect alcohols in moderation. The type of alcohol you choose has a profound effect on your health and how you feel the next day.

BULLETPROOF BEVERAGES

WATER AND MINERAL WATER

Water is obviously important to keep you hydrated and alive. Your body needs water throughout the day, and it can only absorb it at a slow rate. It's far better to drink half a glass several times a day than it is to drink a large amount in one sitting. Don't worry about drinking eight glasses of water a day; instead focus on honoring your thirst and always drink a glass of water after you urinate. Speaking of that, it's not a good idea to look at the color of your urine to determine how hydrated you are. Many people think clear urine is a sign of good hydration, but this probably means you either drank way too much water, which disrupts your electrolytes, or that you ate something toxic and your body is trying to dilute it so it does less damage to your kidneys and bladder. If you listen to your body and drink water throughout the day, yellow pee is fine.

BULLETPROOF COFFEE

This almost goes without saying, but Bulletproof Coffee is the most Bulletproof beverage you can drink in the morning. You've already read about how plain untested coffee beans are Kryptonite because of mold toxins and how some special types of beans are Suspect because they're less likely to have toxins but are untested. Using beans that have been tested to show they have virtually no toxins is a huge upgrade. The addition of grass-fed butter and Brain Octane Oil is like icing on the Bulletproof Coffee cake.

HIGH-QUALITY GREEN TEA
OR YERBA MATTE

Green tea can provide antioxidant and anti-inflammatory benefits as long as you buy a quality brand. Green tea has a ton of antioxidants, but it can deplete folate levels, especially in pregnant women. Green tea extract has also been shown to lower testosterone in one controversial study,[27] and consuming too much green tea can provide unhealthy levels of fluoride. This is a healthy beverage, and you can blend butter and Brain Octane Oil into it if you like, but I recommend you stick to one or two cups a day at most.

COCONUT MILK

For all the same reasons that coconut oil is so great for your body and your performance, coconut milk is, too. There are two things to watch out for, however. One is that some coconut milk companies use carrageenan as an emulsifier, which can damage the lining of the gut. Others use guar gum, which is acceptable, but not as healthy as using no emulsifier at all. The other problem is BPA, the plasticizer that is estrogenic and lines most cans. Look online to find a list of BPA-free brands. If you want your coconut milk to taste even more like cream, try blending in a little grass-fed butter! Beware—light coconut milk is a scam. All they do is add water to coconut milk. Regular coconut milk can be quite thick, so try diluting it a bit with water yourself.

SUSPECT BEVERAGES

COCONUT WATER

While coconut milk is full of healthy fats, coconut water is mostly sugar. It does have some nutritional benefits, but it will take you out of fat-burning mode and might cause food cravings later. You'll get better results if you only drink it once in a while after a workout or before bed.

HERBAL TEA/UNSWEETENED ICED TEA

Herbal tea is fine, but it doesn't provide the same health benefits as green tea, and it's important to pay attention to which herbs were used. Most herbal teas have medicinal effects, so be aware of the impact of those herbs on how you feel. Even something as simple as mint tea may improve your digestion, but cause a food craving for you. This could happen with any tea if it has flavoring additives or if you're sensitive to any of the ingredients. High-quality teas are less likely to contain additives that will cause food cravings.

BOTTLED NUT MILKS

Nut milks have the same problems as nuts but are often worse because the bottled nut milks are made from nuts that are too ugly to sell. What makes nuts ugly? You guessed it—damage to the nuts, which opens the door for mold to invade. Some companies also press the oils from nuts and then use the waste products to make "nut milks," so make sure to choose a high-quality brand. Like with coconut milk, avoid brands that use carrageenan, an emulsifier that is irritating, weakening, and willpower sapping.

VODKA, GIN, TEQUILA, AND WHISKEY

These alcohols have the lowest amounts of sugar and antinutrients—the two things that make most alcoholic drinks Kryptonite. But don't be fooled into thinking that you can drink unlimited amounts of these and still perform at your best. Alcohol will almost always inhibit performance and lead to brain fog, so this is one case where moderation is extremely important. Of course, you should be mindful of what you mix your alcohol with. Try drinking vodka with soda water and a squeeze of lemon or lime instead of adding fructose bombs like juice or Kryptonite prepackaged mixers to your drink.

DRY CHAMPAGNE AND DRY WHITE WINE

These are even more suspect than the liquors mentioned above because they are unfiltered and contain more fungal metabolites. However, these are much safer than red wine or beer, which I discuss below. It's best to save these for a special occasion.

FRESHLY SQUEEZED FRUIT JUICE

These are too high in damaging fructose to consume regularly, but they won't hurt your performance too much as long as they are freshly squeezed, don't contain any added sugars or fillers, and you only have them once in a while. To be sure of this, it's best to squeeze them yourself. But keep in mind that one glass of fruit juice is likely to push you over your limit of 25 grams of fructose a day.

KRYPTONITE BEVERAGES

SOY MILK

Soy milk is Kryptonite for the same reasons as other soy products, but it's quite possibly the worst one. Like nut milks, soy milk is often made from lower-quality soy that's more likely to have mold from field or storage practices. There are nine kinds of toxin-forming fungus that impact soy crops in the United States alone.[28] Try diluted coconut milk instead.

WHITE AND RED WINE

Many people think wine is a health food, but it simply isn't true. The wine industry has done a great job of telling us that resveratrol, a compound found in grapes, is good for us. Whether this is true or not is still a matter of debate. (I believe it's probably a useful supplement.) But what is not up for debate is the fact that wine has such low amounts of resveratrol that it doesn't matter whether or not it's beneficial. You'd have to drink hundreds of bottles of wine to get the benefits of a couple capsules of resveratrol.

We actually still know very little about the effects of resveratrol on humans; studies have shown it may disrupt hormones.[29] Meanwhile, wine is full of unfiltered yeast, which triggers yeast growth and brain fog, and histamine, which will give you headaches, brain fog, and a spare tire. One of the biggest problems with red wine in particular is the presence of the mold toxin ochratoxin A, especially in American wine, which is not subject to the strict European standards of 2 parts per billion. Red wine has higher levels than white because mold forms on the outside of the fruit, and more skin contact time is required to extract the pigments and tannins in red wine compared to white.[30]

It's up to you to decide whether the pleasures of wine are worth the documented toxins and your resulting decline in performance.

BEER

Tragically, beer has the most toxins of any common alcoholic beverage. Drinking beer will wreck your performance, cause terrible food cravings, and make it extremely difficult for you to lose weight. Plus, beer has all the grain toxins and more ochratoxin than wine or untested coffee. They don't call it a beer belly for nothing.

SODA AND OTHER SWEETENED DRINKS

Soda is a massive source of high-fructose corn syrup, which causes enormous food cravings, and phosphoric acid, which weakens your bones. There is no place in your diet for naturally sweetened soda or its even more dangerous cousin, diet soda, which causes more intense food cravings because of its artificial sweeteners. If you like the sensation of drinking something carbonated, try sparkling water with lemon or lime. My favorite is unsweetened San Pellegrino water.

SPORTS DRINKS

These major sources of high-fructose corn syrup are basically soda with artificial colorings and no carbonation. Sports drinks simply don't have a place in a healthy diet, and they'll do far more harm to your athletic performance than good. If you're participating in a high-endurance sport, try drinking water with a bit of added sea salt instead.

It's true that variety is the spice of life, and having a variety of flavors to create your meals with is important not just for adding flavor, but also for creating happiness. By choosing your spices carefully, you can create a huge difference in how you feel all day long. This is especially true when it comes to food cravings. I was shocked to discover how the quality of spices I used impacted how I felt and the fact that artificial sweeteners and flavor enhancers were so harmful to my cognitive performance. The good news is that there are some flavorings like turmeric, oregano, and even vanilla that are not only neutral, but actually beneficial. In terms of getting natural polyphenols that are good for gut bacteria, it's hard to beat herbs and spices. It's just important to use high-quality versions of the right ones and store them properly.

CHAPTER 12

THE WAY YOU COOK YOUR FOOD CAN MAKE IT TOXIC

hether you're an accomplished chef or someone who's used to getting takeout every night, it can be intimidating to prepare new meals when starting any diet. I've taken the guesswork out of this by creating recipes (see page 253) that range from extremely simple combinations of Bulletproof ingredients to more labor-intensive gourmet meals. You can choose to prepare and eat anywhere within this range, but first it's important to understand what different cooking methods actually do to your food.

As you read earlier, when I started to build the Bulletproof Diet, one of the primary goals was to eliminate inflammation from all sources. During my time as a raw vegan, I learned quite a lot about toxins that are formed in food during certain cooking methods. When I put it all together, it became painfully obvious that the way I processed and cooked my food (particularly proteins and fats) played a large role in my body's level of inflammation. I started studying modernist cuisine with its different cooking methods, and instead of using its scientifically accurate measurements and precision to target flavor alone, I aimed for the meals that made me feel the best. It worked, and revealed quite clearly which cooking methods reduce inflammation and which ones caused it.

This is why how you cook your food is just as important as what you eat on the Bulletproof Diet. When smoking, frying, or grilling meat, two carcinogens are produced: heterocyclic amines (HCAs) and polycyclic aromatic hydrocarbons (PAHs). HCAs are formed when amino acids, sugars, and creatine react at high temperatures. PAHs are formed when the fat and juices from meat are burned in the flames of an open fire (such as when grilling) and then adhere to the surface of the meat. Two other sources of PAHs are car exhaust fumes and cigarette smoke. That's right—grilling your meat can be as damaging to your body as smoking! When cooked above about 320°F, all meat produces some of these carcinogenic compounds. The amount

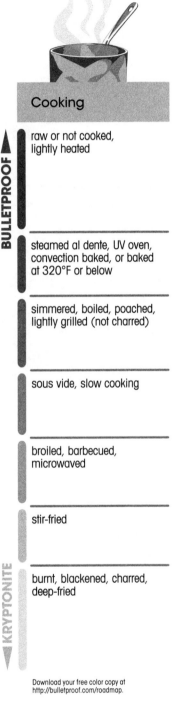

Cooking

BULLETPROOF ▲

raw or not cooked, lightly heated

steamed al dente, UV oven, convection baked, or baked at 320°F or below

simmered, boiled, poached, lightly grilled (not charred)

sous vide, slow cooking

broiled, barbecued, microwaved

stir-fried

▼ KRYPTONITE

burnt, blackened, charred, deep-fried

Download your free color copy at http://bulletproof.com/roadmap.

depends on the temperature, how long the meat is cooked, the spices used, and the actual cooking method.

Another problem with some cooking methods is that they damage proteins. Denatured proteins, which have lost their structure due to heat, aren't toxic in and of themselves. But the more heated a protein is, the more denatured it gets and the less likely it is that your body will be able to take advantage of its signaling molecules. For example, research in mice has shown that only whey protein that hasn't been denatured boosts glutathione, the body's master antioxidant.[1] This is why I cook my proteins as little as possible.

The final problem with some cooking methods is that they oxidize fats. Fats are your friends, and it's important to be nice to them! As you know, polyunsaturated fats are highly reactive to heat and other chemical stressors. When heated, these oils produce compounds called dicarbonyls that cause cell mutations and may contribute to cancer.[2]

Before you start cooking your Bulletproof meals, you need to know which cooking methods will create these toxins in your food. To simplify things, here is a list of Bulletproof, Suspect, and Kryptonite cooking methods, organized in order from the safest to the most dangerous, so that you can avoid damaging your precious foods by cooking them the wrong way.

BULLETPROOF COOKING METHODS

RAW

The most Bulletproof way to prepare a fat and most protein is to not cook it. This might strike you as a little odd since lots of your calories on the Bulletproof Diet come from animal products, but grass-fed animal products are much less likely to contain parasites, pathogens, and toxins than those from grain-fed animals, so I think it's safe to eat them on the rare side. Think about adding a raw egg to a smoothie or eating more sushi (without soy sauce) or carpaccio. Most cooking methods also oxidize delicate omega-3 and omega-6 fats, making them inflammatory. This is why a lot of my recipes instruct you to add the fat after you cook the protein or vegetable to keep the fats raw.

LIGHTLY HEATED

If you're cooking meat, the best method is to place it in a small amount of water (to protect against oxidation and save the fats/juices) on low to medium heat (to avoid damaging proteins and destroying nutrients), tightly covered or for a short duration (to avoid oxidizing fats). Whatever method you're using, make sure to use the least amount of heat you can to get it cooked and still make it taste good.

STEAMED AL DENTE

Steaming is one of the safest cooking methods for meat and the best one for most vegetables. It saves most of the nutrients in your food from damage, makes vegetables and meats more palatable, and allows you to make a greater variety of dishes. However, steaming can easily be overdone. Steaming your vegetables into mush might make them easier to eat, but it also destroys many of their nutrients.

BAKED AT 320°F OR BELOW

Baking tends to be a riskier cooking method because of the high temperatures and available oxygen. Heating sugars (even the ones in plants) at high temperatures for a long time can produce AGEs and free radicals, while baking proteins can damage the protein bonds and cause the formation of toxic glutamate. Baking fats causes them to oxidize. All of these reactions cause inflammation, which decreases your mental and physical performance, but baking at temperatures below 320°F reduces the risks. Try adding turmeric, green tea, lemon, rosemary, sage, or oregano to protect the fats in your food from oxidation, too.

BOILED OR POACHED

Boiling water prevents oxidation of fats and protein because it displaces most of the oxygen. Boiled meat often isn't particularly flavorful, but it's fine for soups and shredded meat dishes. Boiled vegetables are healthy, and the extra water you drain away may remove unwanted antinutrients.

SUSPECT COOKING METHODS

SIMMERED

Simmering helps prevent fats from oxidizing, but it does tend to fully denature proteins. Simmering for a short period of time is fine, but leaving a bunch of meat on the stove to simmer for hours is not a good idea. Simmering is also a good option for vegetables as long as you don't overcook them.

SOUS VIDE

This method of cooking food in a water bath can make meat literally melt in your mouth. I've had a sous vide setup in my kitchen for a decade. It's a great cooking method, but it does have a few downsides. The main risk is that BPA and other compounds can leach into your food from the plastic bags you use. The best way to avoid this problem is to use a glass jar packed fully, instead. Just about every recipe you'll find for sous vide pays little attention to the biological effects of the cooking method. We honestly don't know what you get when you cook an artichoke at 160°F for 10 hours. Did you make it safer for consumption or less safe? Did the meat you cooked for 12 hours make it hot enough to prevent bacterial degradation and histamine? This is a fun way of cooking that produces amazing culinary results. See how you feel when cooking this way.

LIGHTLY GRILLED (NOT CHARRED)

This gives meat an unmistakable flavor and texture while keeping toxin formation to a minimum. The best way to grill your meat is so that the outside is just barely browned but the inside is still medium-rare to rare. This reduces the formation of toxins caused by charring meat while still giving your meat that wonderful grilled flavor and texture.

SLOW COOKING

Slow cooking is an easy and time-efficient way to prepare meals, but it does have a few downsides. Long, slow cooking breaks down collagen, making for soft, delicious meat dishes. However, it can also produce glutamate and overcook meat. Keep it tightly covered and use lots of antioxidant spices like turmeric and rosemary, and consider adding some ascorbic acid (vitamin C) powder if you're planning to simmer something for several hours.

BROILED

Broiling uses high heat from all sides to brown meat, which denatures the proteins more than the Bulletproof cooking methods. Broiling also oxidizes fats and causes glutamate to form outside the meat while destroying more nutrients in your food than other cooking methods. It's okay to make a broiled dish every now and then, but it shouldn't be your default cooking method.

KRYPTONITE COOKING METHODS

BARBECUED

While barbecuing meat over an open flame or grill makes it taste great, it also causes a few serious problems. When the fats hit the coals, they form cancer- and inflammation-causing HCAs and PAHs. Most barbecue sauces have sugar and MSG, too. In most cases, you can get a similar taste and texture from low-temperature grilling, which produces fewer performance-robbing toxins, and by making your own Bulletproof barbecue sauce.

BURNT, BLACKENED, OR CHARRED

Burning, blackening, or charring meat oxidizes the fat molecules, making them inflammatory. Oxidized fats also disrupt hormonal signaling, which can make you less sensitive to insulin, and thus, fatter. These methods also denature proteins, which makes them irritating to your immune system and harder to digest. They also produce mutagenic and carcinogenic substances. Finally, these cooking methods produce glutamate, a neurotransmitter that in large amounts overexcites brain cells to death. All of these things decrease your mental and physical performance and may even make you age faster. Never eat blackened meat.

DEEP-FRIED

Deep-frying is one of the worst ways to cook your food, as it bathes your food in oxidized fats, denatured proteins, and glycated sugars. The high temperatures used during deep-frying produce a number of toxic compounds that may increase your risk of cancer.

MICROWAVED

Microwaved food is fully denatured, and one (albeit controversial) study showed that microwaves cause changes in HDL, LDL, and white blood cells.[3] Microwave ovens also tend to create high amounts of electromagnetic fields in your kitchen. I don't recommend using them.

LOSE A POUND A DAY WITHOUT BEING HUNGRY: THE 2-WEEK BULLETPROOF PROTOCOL

O ver the course of developing the Bulletproof Diet, I switched from one diet to another several times. I found that each time, it took about 2 weeks to settle into a new diet and get used to the difference you can feel in your body as it adjusts to receiving very different foods. Over the next 2 weeks, your brain and body are going to become Bulletproof. As you remove antinutrients from your diet and begin eating the most nutritious, satisfying foods that exist, your brain will feel noticeably sharper and your energy will skyrocket. While you're enjoying plenty of delicious healthy fats, proteins, and vegetables, you'll lose up to a pound a day without the sense of deprivation and cravings you probably expect from any diet. Your skin will glow, your hair will strengthen, and you'll wake up with a new spring in your step, more ready than ever to take on the day and whatever it holds.

Some people have told me that losing weight so effortlessly while eating foods like steak and butter that they previously thought of as sinful felt "wrong." One well-known publishing executive went off the Bulletproof Diet after 6 months because he "got tired of never feeling hungry." But the combination of better focus and easy weight loss on the Bulletproof Diet is what makes it so right. This is how you were meant to eat, and now you can take control of your body and enjoy reaping the results of controlling your own biology.

The first step to following the Bulletproof Diet is to get rid of all the Kryptonite foods in your house. Take an hour to go through your fridge and your pantry and throw all the garbage like chips, cookies, packaged foods, sodas, margarines, artificial sweeteners, breads, and crackers where they belong—in the trash. These foods are not good for you, and you don't need to have them sitting around the house sapping your willpower. Keeping this stuff around will only make it easier for your Labrador brain to hijack your human brain and cause you to have "just one bite." And while eating one or two cookies or pretzels may not seem like a big deal, one or two will lead to food cravings later that cause you to eat the whole bag.

Do you remember the old Lay's potato chip ad campaign that said, "Bet you can't eat just one"? Well, they were right. That ad was actually completely truthful. You can't eat just one because those foods are designed to be addictive. Cleaning out your cupboards will keep you from having to use up your willpower saying no to the Kryptonite lurking behind every corner, and it will give you a fresh start to becoming Bulletproof. We're going to turn off those food cravings by eliminating toxins and increasing fat, but removing temptation will make the first few days a lot easier.

As a professional athlete and a health-care professional, I have implemented the Bulletproof lifestyle and felt the physical, psychological, and spiritual effects almost immediately. I am so passionate about the benefits of the Bulletproof lifestyle that I feel obliged to tell my fellow athletes, colleagues, friends, and family about it so they, too, can increase their human life performance. **—Josh Binstock, Olympic beach volleyball athlete and chiropractor**

> The biggest change from the Bulletproof Diet was not what I took away but what I added. Fat! This, of course, started with Bulletproof Coffee and Intermittent Fasting. Within a week, I noticed the lack of bloating and the reduction in hunger. Now 10 weeks in, I've lost 20 pounds, my creativity is off the charts, and I have real energy to take control of my life's activities.
> —Laura

Once your house is free of the Kryptonite foods that will make you weak and fat and limit your performance, it's time to restock your kitchen, but this time with delicious, satisfying Bulletproof foods. Use the Bulletproof Diet Roadmap as a guide, focusing on Bulletproof foods and avoiding the Suspect and Kryptonite ingredients that call to you from the center aisles. You can also download a free shopping guide at the Bulletproof Executive Web site. Suffice it to say, your shopping cart should be full of vegetables along with plenty of healthy fats and proteins. Then add a few Bulletproof starches and fruits and your choice of flavorings. If your shopping cart isn't mostly green, you haven't bought enough veggies—go back and get some more.

Many people don't consider shopping for food online, but I think this is a great way to research different brands and exact ingredients before making a purchase. Local farmers' markets or community-supported agriculture shares are the best sources of local, organic, sustainable vegetables, and they often have great options for animal products, too. If you don't have those options near you, try a combination of online shopping and the best items you can find at your local grocery store. Just make sure to fill up your kitchen with as many Bulletproof foods as you can to avoid being tempted by quick fixes and fast food.

TRACKING YOUR KRYPTONITE

Food sensitivities are the result of either an immune-system reaction to certain foods or the body's lack of proper enzymes to digest them. When the body reacts to a food, it sends out inflammatory proteins and cortisol, which create low-level chronic inflammation. This type of chronic inflammation may impair digestion and cause sore joints, headaches, food cravings, and brain fog. Inflammation also triggers weight gain because it affects a specific part of the brain (the hypothalamus), causing it to become insulin and leptin resistant. Decreasing inflammation is critical in any effective fat-loss protocol, including the Bulletproof Diet. Unfortunately, most people with low-level chronic inflammation do not connect the symptoms with the foods that are causing them.

Because of your individual biochemistry, you respond to every food you eat differently than the mythical "average person." Some foods, like gluten and margarine, are Kryptonite for everyone, but even those have a bigger impact on some people than others. Suspect foods will either work for you or they won't, in which case they're Kryptonite for *you*. The red bell pepper, for example, is a Suspect food that makes some people feel great, but triggers arthritic pain in others. When a specific food is Kryptonite for you but not for others, it means you have a food sensitivity or allergy to that particular food.

The fastest way to get a pretty complete list of your food sensitivities is to drop about $350 by going to your doctor and asking for an IgG/IgE blood panel testing for food allergies. You'll get a report listing the foods that you're sensitive to—your list of personal Kryptonite. The only limitation is that there are some immunity-based food sensitivities that cause white blood cell proliferation even when there are no antibodies to a food, and allergy blood tests will not detect those sensitivities. Still, if you can afford the test, this data is priceless.

GETTING THE MOST FROM YOUR TWO MEALS A DAY

Because you'll be doing Bulletproof Intermittent Fasting while on the 2-Week Protocol, your breakfast each day will be delicious, satisfying

Bulletproof Coffee. This will turn off hunger and cravings, give you a huge boost of energy in the morning, and fuel your brain and your body. If you make it with the Brain Octane Oil that produces four times as many ketones as plain coconut oil does, it can help you enter ketosis faster and burn fat while working with increased focus and attention right through until lunch.

If you're a woman over 40, or need to lose a lot of weight, and/or you're not satisfied by Bulletproof Coffee alone, it's a good idea to add 25 to 30 grams of protein. I recommend drinking Bulletproof Coffee with added grass-fed collagen protein. When you use the Brain Octane oil, it's possible to have ketones present to fuel your brain while the protein will help stabilize your leptin levels to ensure long-term success. If you use plain coconut oil, it's tasty, but it's not all the way Bulletproof, as you'll have fewer ketones and may feel less energy, but you should still feel no hunger.

For the rest of the day, you'll focus on eating two meals with massive amounts of vegetables, lots of healthy fats, moderate amounts of protein, and, during and after dinner, small amounts of starch. Remember that to get the best results with Bulletproof Intermittent Fasting, you should consume both meals within about a 6-hour window. This means that if your dinner is at 7:00 p.m., you shouldn't eat lunch the next day until 1:00 p.m. If you normally eat dinner later, your lunches should be later, too. You don't have to do this exactly right to reap the benefits, but the more often you limit your feeding window to 6 hours or less, the more you'll benefit. You'll get a better reduction in inflammation and an even bigger boost in energy and brainpower. But don't skip a meal just because you missed the window.

Once a week (on days 6 and 13), you'll get to try out Bulletproof Protein Fasting. To get a thorough scrub-down of your cells that will help you feel, look, and think like a much younger person, it's important to stick to the program on these days and limit your protein intake by eating the recommended meals. This is also your opportunity to re-feed on carbohy-

> A little over a year ago, I was over 230 pounds, all-around physically and mentally unhealthy, and had little to motivate me. Now I'm lighter, more on top of things, sober, and my productivity levels are at the highest they've ever been. The switch was flipped on when I first started listening to the Bulletproof podcast and was inspired and empowered by so many intelligent individuals giving insight about how to perfect the art of life.
> **—Mark Heylmun, lead guitarist, Suicide Silence**

drates, and I've focused the meal plan for those days to include the most beneficial Bulletproof high-carb, low-protein meals.

You may be accustomed to using snacks to temporarily satisfy your hunger because you're eating less satiating foods at mealtime, but this backfires by stimulating your appetite. Eating two or three large meals instead of grazing throughout the day minimizes the release of hunger hormones and keeps you satiated instead of prolonging your hunger when you nibble on small bites. This is one of the ways the Bulletproof Diet hacks hunger, and as a result, snacks are no longer temptations on the Bulletproof Diet. You simply won't care about them because your Labrador brain will know it isn't starving.

If you follow the meal plan closely, you shouldn't need snacks because you'll be resilient enough to go more than 5 hours between meals without losing energy. I now see a snack craving as a sign that I'm doing something wrong. One of the most important things I've learned as a biohacker is that hunger is almost completely controllable. On the Bulletproof Diet, you won't feel the same type of desperate hunger that you did before. You'll sense when it's time for a meal and feel like you can eat, but you won't be nearly as ravenous.

If you do find yourself wanting a snack between meals while following the 2-week plan, it's probably because you're used to taking a break to eat and not because of actual physical hunger. If this happens, try taking a break from work. Do some deep breathing or take a 10-minute walk. If that doesn't do the trick, it's okay to eat something, but make sure it's a high-fat snack that will satisfy you rather than a typical high-carb snack food. It might also be because your previous meal wasn't large enough. That's okay. Here are a few ideas for Bulletproof Snacks:

- More Bulletproof Coffee (as long as it's before 2:00 p.m.)
- 1 tablespoon of butter mixed with chocolate powder
- Bulletproof Guacamole with celery and/or cucumber slices
- Very dark—90 percent cocoa—high-quality chocolate from Europe
- Almond butter (if it agrees with you) on celery sticks
- Equal parts almond butter (if it agrees with you) and grass-fed butter mixed with cocoa powder for a chocolaty flavor— spread it on veggies or just eat it by the spoonful! Almond butter with cocoa powder alone tastes amazing, but it doesn't have enough saturated fat. Adding butter solves this problem beautifully. You can even add grass-fed butter to almond butter when eating it with celery sticks to add a healthy fat and nutrient boost.

2-WEEK PROTOCOL

For your first 2 weeks on the Bulletproof Diet, I've taken all of the guess-work out of what you should eat each day. This will make it easy for you to make these important changes to your diet while focusing on how

A number of years ago, Dave Asprey helped me recover from hypothyroidism by changing my diet. With his help, I effortlessly lost 50 pounds in 3 months and became much healthier. He's a brain and body hacker extraordinaire. —**Steve** amazing you feel and the incredible differences in how you look! Simply choose a meal from the list of options and see the recipe Appendix for detailed instructions.

Keep in mind that I'm intentionally leaving out specific portion sizes. Your portion size should be based on what your body wants, and it will self-regulate depending how you slept, the weather, what you did that day, and your metabolism. Eat until you're full. It's time to trust your body to regulate its own energy.

Over the next 2 weeks, you should enjoy your first taste of high performance and power. You'll feel a huge difference as your body sheds toxins along with weight, and you should lose up to a pound a day by eating from the following food plan. Each day, you'll pick one item from each of the lunch, dinner, and dessert lists below. Yes, you get to eat dessert—every day if you want to, although these are not desserts you'll find at the store. There are enough options here so that you'll have plenty of variety and never feel deprived. Some of these meals are extremely easy and fast to prepare, such as the Smoked Salmon and Avocado "Not-Sushi" and Smoked Salmon Butter Bites, while others take more time and effort. Take a close look at the recipes in the Appendix before selecting your meals for the first 2 weeks so you know what you'll need to prepare.

Day 6 and day 13 of your first 2 weeks will be your protein fast days. On these days, simply choose from the list of Bulletproof Protein Fast meals instead of the regular meal list. Yes, this will take a little effort and planning, but the amazing anti-inflammatory and energy-boosting results will be well worth it!

BULLETPROOF MEAL PLAN

Here are the delicious meals you'll be enjoying for the next 2 weeks. Each day, simply choose one meal from each category to begin feeling, looking, and performing better than ever.

Bulletproof Breakfast

(Choose one to be eaten as soon as you get up or whenever you are accustomed to eating breakfast.)

- Bulletproof Coffee (page 253)
  (*Note:* If you are a woman over 40 or are significantly overweight, try adding grass-fed collagen to your Bulletproof Coffee or even eating a little protein after your coffee.)
- No-Coffee Vanilla Latte (for those who don't like or can't drink coffee; page 254)
- Green tea blended with butter and Brain Octane Oil (This is not as powerful as Bulletproof Coffee, however!)

Bulletproof Lunches

(Choose one to be eaten 15 to 18 hours after last night's dinner.)

- Smoked Salmon and Avocado "Not-Sushi" (page 255)
- Smoked Salmon Butter Bites (page 255)
- Bulletproof Poached Eggs with Sautéed Greens (page 256)
- Bulletproof Taco Salad (page 257)
- Bulletproof Meatballs (page 258)
- Bulletproof One-Pot Soup (page 258)
- Bulletproof Un-Omelet (page 259)
- Upgraded Kale Shake (page 260)
- Bulletproof Benedict (page 261)

Bulletproof Dinners

(Choose one to be eaten 5 to 6 hours after lunch.)

- Bulletproof Hash (page 262)
- Roasted Pork Belly with Vegetables (page 263)
- Bulletproof Roast with Brussels Sprouts (page 264)

- Bulletproof Stew (page 265)
- Roasted Lamb Rack with Vegetables (page 266)
- Bulletproof Pulled Something! (page 267) with a vegetable side dish from the list below
- Ground beef wrapped in bacon with a vegetable side dish from the list that follows
- Bulletproof Baked Fish (page 268) with a vegetable side dish from the list below

Bulletproof Vegetable Side Dishes

- Sautéed Greens (page 256)
- Cauliflower-Bacon Mash (page 268)
- "Cheesy" Butternut Squash (page 269)
- Creamed Vegetables (page 269)
- Lime-Cilantro Cauliflower "Not-Rice" (page 270)
- Baked Broccoli with Turmeric + Ginger (page 270)

Bulletproof Desserts

(Choose one to be eaten right after dinner.)

- Shockingly Rich Chocolate Truffle Pudding (page 280)
- Almond Truffle Cups (page 280)
- Coconut-Blueberry Ultimately Creamy Panna Cotta (page 281)
- Creamy Coconut "Get Some" Ice Cream (page 282)
- Bulletproof Cupcakes (page 283)

BULLETPROOF PROTEIN FAST MEAL PLAN

On day 6 and day 13, the following meals will help your body detox even more efficiently while giving you an extra boost of energy.

Bulletproof Protein Fast Breakfast

(Choose one to have as soon as you get up or whenever you are accustomed to eating breakfast.)

- Bulletproof Coffee (without any added protein; page 253)
- No-Coffee Vanilla Latte (for those who don't like or can't drink coffee; page 254)
- Green tea blended with butter and MCT oil (This is not as powerful as Bulletproof Coffee, however!)

Bulletproof Protein Fast Lunches

(Choose one to be eaten 15 to 18 hours after last night's dinner.)

- Upgraded Kale Shake (page 260)
- Upgraded Guacamole (page 278) with cucumber and/or celery slices
- Bulletproof Sweet Potato–Ginger Soup (page 271)
- Upgraded Iceberg Salad (page 272) with Baked Carrot Fries (page 274)

Bulletproof Protein Fast Dinners

(Choose one to be eaten 5 to 6 hours after lunch.)

- Upgraded Iceberg Salad (page 272) with Lemon Rice (page 276)
- Bulletproof Bean-Free Dahl and Rice (page 275)
- Bulletproof Carrot-Fennel Soup with Rice (page 276)
- Baked Sweet Potatoes (page 277) with Upgraded Guacamole (page 278)

Bulletproof Protein Fast Desserts

(Choose one to be eaten soon after dinner.)

- Coconut-Blueberry Ultimately Creamy Panna Cotta (page 280)
- Bulletproof Berry Bowl (page 284)

TROUBLESHOOTING THE BULLETPROOF DIET

If you follow the meal plan closely, you should feel fantastic for the next 2 weeks, but if the going gets tough, there are two likely culprits. If you've been on a low-fat, low-calorie, or vegan diet, your Labrador brain knows your body is so starved for precious healthy fats that it will tell you to overeat them. The problem is that it takes your body anywhere from a week to a month to fully turn on its fat-digestion systems if they've been lying fallow. When you eat too much fat before your body is ready to use it, the result is what Bulletproof fans call "disaster pants"—not exactly the performance boost you were looking for! MCT oil has the strongest influence on disaster pants; it's powerful stuff. The shortest chain C8 MCT in Brain Octane Oil causes less disaster pants and provides more brain energy. Go slow when adding Brain Octane Oil to your coffee. Start with as little as 1 teaspoon of Brain Octane Oil and increase from there. More is not always better!

Whether or not you experience disaster pants, you'll get the best results when you teach your body to use fat as fuel. You do this by taking digestive enzymes that contain fat-digesting lipase and betaine HCl, which help your body have enough stomach acid to use fat and protein. Most adults are somewhat deficient in stomach acid. For most people, taking these supplements before or during (but *not* after) a meal solves the fat-digestion problem. It may take a few weeks, but your body will get used to using fat for fuel, so you won't need them forever. They do provide ongoing benefits, so you may choose to keep using them. Some people don't need them at all.

Another possible issue is acid reflux, which is the result of the valve at the top of your stomach closing improperly because it didn't get the right signal. Keep in mind that the signal for this valve to close is stomach acid! Many people think stomach acid causes indigestion, but the opposite is actually true. It's weak stomach acid that leaves the valve open, leading to indigestion. This is something integrative medical practitioners have known for years. I once had severe heartburn that a doctor treated with a proton pump inhibitor that may have contributed to food allergies I later developed. Sure enough, the heartburn went away when I took betaine HCl. It turns out that this supplement that solves the fat-digestion problem by increasing stomach acid can fix acid reflux, too. If you try this and the pain gets worse, no big deal—taking a tiny amount of baking soda to neutralize the acid is okay, too. It's not a good idea to always rely on baking soda because you need stomach acid to digest properly, but it will help in a pinch so you can experience all the benefits of the Bulletproof Diet.

BULLETPROOF FOR LIFE

After following the 2-week plan, I hope and trust that you're starting to see the pounds come off while also noticing a difference in your energy level, focus, and performance. The first thing I suggest you do after 2 weeks on the Bulletproof Diet is to go out and eat a huge pizza, Chinese food, or whatever nutritional Kryptonite you craved the most over the past 2 weeks. Wash it down with some beer or red wine. This sounds crazy, doesn't it? But now that you've gotten a taste of what it feels like to be Bulletproof, it's time to show yourself the difference in how you feel, look, and perform when you go back to eating Kryptonite. Does it make you feel sluggish, tired, bloated, and unfocused? Do your pants feel a little tighter from the inflammation? Are you suddenly craving sugar like crazy even though you just ate? The truth is that this is what your food was doing to you all the time before you started to become Bulletproof, but it was barely noticeable because you felt this way all the time. The only difference is that now you know there's another way.

When I started down this path, I allowed myself a cheat day once a week, but I soon found that the cost in how it made me feel the rest of the week wasn't worth it. Why spend half the week recovering from your cheat day when you can make better choices and spend the whole week feeling awesome? When I ate Kryptonite on the weekends, Monday and Tuesday weren't good days for me, and I finally realized that life is too precious to spend 2 days a week feeling less energy just so I could enjoy some foods. The best thing to do is to find foods that you enjoy that also make you feel awesome. That's what this is all about.

You have the choice to go back to this low level of performance or to make Bulletproof your new standard so you can perform at your best all day, every day. If you choose that path, this is only the beginning. You'll continue to lose weight and feel great while enjoying nutritious, rich Bulletproof foods. As you learn to navigate the Bulletproof Diet Roadmap, you'll find other foods that are compatible with your system and add those to the menu. No matter what you choose to eat, it's somewhere on the roadmap. Where do you want to be?

Being Bulletproof for life doesn't mean being forever limited to the 2-week meal plan or even the list of Bulletproof foods. It's about maintaining your results by making better—but not perfect—choices most of the time. With this book, you have all of the information you need to get the results you want. Every time you choose what food to eat, you can decide whether to have something that will boost your performance or something that will make you weak and sap your willpower. Being Bulletproof isn't black-and-white; it's a wide spectrum. The more Bulletproof foods you eat, the better you'll look and feel, while the more Kryptonite you eat, the more prone you'll be to weight gain, a short temper, and brain fog. It's that simple.

You may not know it, but you've always been on the Bulletproof Diet. You may have just made poorer choices in the past and eaten more

Kryptonite than you have been for the past 2 weeks, but that's because you didn't have a roadmap or a tool to help you navigate it. From now on, every meal is an opportunity to make better choices that will boost your performance and make you more Bulletproof.

In maintenance mode, the three variables you can play around with are how many Suspect foods you eat, how often you visit the sketchy neighborhoods on the roadmap (starches, nuts, and fruits), and how often you do Bulletproof Intermittent Fasting. If you want, try eating a few more carbs in the evening, and if your pants get tight, simply cut back. You might even have starch in the morning sometimes if you really want to, as you now know your body is resilient and can handle it. I don't get a lot of fresh fruits where I live, so if I go on a trip to a fruit-growing region in the peak of summer, I definitely go over 25 grams of fructose a day, and I don't feel bad about it. This might result in a few extra food cravings, but I understand the risks and make my choices accordingly. When I start to gain a few pounds and want to shed them, I cut back on fruits and save them for dessert.

If it makes you feel good while you're in maintenance mode, you can eat something for breakfast besides Bulletproof Coffee and do Bulletproof Intermittent Fasting only occasionally, but Bulletproof Intermittent Fasting is so painless and so much easier than cooking and eating breakfast that you may prefer to stick to Bulletproof Intermittent Fasting 7 days a week. Frankly, I don't really enjoy breakfast unless it's something wonderful like high-quality bacon and duck eggs. Otherwise, I feel better when I

The diet is great. I've been doing it for about 8 months now. At 5 foot 11, I was 180 and looking to simply remove those midlife love handles and 10 pounds. I already work out 5 days a week for about 4 years now, and still couldn't get rid of those things. About 3 months in, the handles are gone and my stomach has serious potential to be chiseled. I now hover at 160 with a target of 165. I couldn't be happier with the changes. **—Jim** just have Bulletproof Coffee. After drinking Bulletproof Coffee for breakfast for 2 weeks, compare how you feel when you eat breakfast, instead, and move forward doing what feels best and gives you the results you want.

Though I no longer have a "cheat day," there are times when I knowingly eat some Kryptonite because I'm willing to take the hit in how I feel. When it's movie night with my family, sometimes I eat popcorn drizzled with grass-fed butter. The next morning, I'm generally not as focused, but . . . it was movie night. Of course, I don't do this when I have a big speaking engagement lined up the next day. You can make the same choices based on what's more important—eating the popcorn (or some other form of Kryptonite) or peak performance the next day. If you have to have some sort of "cheat" food, then have it, and don't think you've fallen off the wagon. Remember, you're still on the diet—you just chose something from the other end of the spectrum. Small variations are fine and do not constitute failure, but of course you'll want to rein it in and stick to Bulletproof foods if you see your weight and performance start to really suffer. If this happens, go back to the 2-week plan to give yourself a refresher course on Bulletproof principles.

In maintenance mode, you'll get the best results from adhering as closely as possible to the main Bulletproof Diet principles—starting the day with Bulletproof Coffee, sticking to Bulletproof Intermittent Fasting on most days, Protein Fasting once a week, and avoiding Kryptonite foods most of the time. The main variable now that you're in maintenance mode is whether you start eating more of the Suspect foods. Different people respond quite differently to the foods on the Bulletproof Diet Roadmap. Based on where their ancestors came from, some people have a genetic capability to break down toxins better than others. If your ancestors came from a potato-producing area such as Ireland, you might be better able to break down the lectins in potatoes than someone whose ancestors came from Asia. But this isn't always the case. Our lineages are often mixed, and many of us don't even have a clear picture of where our ancestors came from.

There may be five Suspect foods that cause you to perform poorly, and if you only eliminate one or two of them you won't feel or look any different. This may cause you to believe that food isn't the variable making you weak and then go forward eating something that is actually hindering you every single day. To complicate this even more, if you are sensitive to certain foods, you may not experience any symptoms right away. Though your body reacts by elevating your heart rate for up to an hour and a half after eating the offending food, it often takes several days before you begin to notice any physical differences. Remember, I saw a 48- to 72-hour lag between the time I consumed gluten and when I started feeling the effects. The exact length of time varies from person to person, but there's often a lag between eating Kryptonite and feeling the effects.

You may do shockingly well on certain Suspect foods, or your performance may suffer. Maybe you're that lucky person that kicks ass while consuming tons of potatoes, but how can you know for sure? The best time to determine which Suspect foods are guilty of destroying your performance is right after completing the 2-week plan. You've just eliminated all Suspect and Kryptonite foods for 2 weeks, so your body is essentially a clean slate. Start adding Suspect foods back into your diet one at a time after completing the 2-week plan. Pay close attention to how you feel. It is worth noting even subtle symptoms like skin rashes, fatigue, or brain fog. This will tell you exactly what foods you are sensitive to and allow you to customize the Bulletproof Diet for even better results.

Once you know which foods you are sensitive to, you are free to go off into the world and make the very best choices for your body and your performance. One of the most challenging places to do this is in a restaurant. Good-quality fats are expensive, so most restaurants are not equipped to serve you a Bulletproof meal that is made of 50 percent healthy fats! Your job is to eat like a king and consume as many healthy fats as you can. But that doesn't mean that you have to stop going out and become a social outcast just when you were starting to look forward to showing off your toned, muscular body. It's easy to make any restaurant meal Bulletproof if you're willing to bring your own "upgrades" and call just a little bit of attention to yourself.

Anytime I go to a restaurant, I bring three things with me: a stick of grass-fed butter, a small container of Brain Octane Oil, and good-quality sea salt. Sometimes I bring an avocado along, too, if the restaurant doesn't serve them. When armed with these three or four items, it's easy to order a basic meal and pump it up to meet your new standards. For breakfast, if I'm not doing Bulletproof Intermittent Fasting I might order poached eggs and then melt my butter on them and pour on the Brain Octane. I've even done this in four-star hotel restaurants. If the chef notices, we always have an interesting conversation.

On the road, I always do Bulletproof Intermittent Fasting because it allows me to go the longest in the morning without thinking about food. To do that, I bring my own beans, which I grind at home before a business trip. Then I ask for a large cup of hot water and add some ground coffee to it. I give it a quick stir, wait a few minutes, and allow the grounds to settle down to the bottom of the cup. Then I decant the black coffee into another cup or my sealable travel mug, add the butter and oil, and either shake or use a tiny battery-powered drink mixer to create my masterpiece. When I do this in coffee shops, people often stop and ask questions, and I'm more than happy to tell them what I'm doing and give them a taste!

This is important—always tip the hardworking person who brings you the hot water. Small coffee shops are not highly profitable, and the people who work there don't make a fortune. You're not using your own beans in their coffee shop to save money; you are doing it because the beans they offer may taste good but are not tested for human performance. Never stiff a barista!

When eating out for lunch or dinner, I pick a wild-caught fish off the menu and ask for a side of steamed vegetables with no sauce. Then I add a chunk of butter to the fish and an entire avocado to the veggies. This helps fill me up and adds calories to the meal without any Kryptonite. Sure, your friends might laugh at you if you do this, but the joke will be

> I don't mean to overstate this, but Bulletproof is saving my life! After a month on the Bulletproof Diet, I feel amazing! Energy levels and productivity are through the roof, mood is great, and hunger and cravings are gone. I spent 3 years at the Ironman distance and never saw my abs. With Bulletproof Coffee for a month with minimal training and one run a week, I can see some definition and feel better than ever! **—Ben**

on them when they see how well your pants start to fit. Remember that you're only going to eat two meals a day, so they need to be large and packed with nutrition.

If there's no high-quality protein on the menu, I sometimes go vegetarian and just order white rice and steamed veggies and add butter, Brain Octane oil, and a whole avocado. Other times I add avocado and Brain Octane oil to a large salad. The most important thing is to avoid restaurant sauces and dressings that so often contain high-fructose corn syrup, bad fats, and/or MSG. I know that if I don't get any protein at one meal I won't starve, but if I accidentally ingest MSG, my performance will certainly suffer.

Making similar choices and prioritizing your performance over convenience is the key to becoming Bulletproof for life. What will you be capable of when you're filled with an energy, determination, and focus that you've never felt before?

CONCLUSION

WHAT TO DO WITH YOUR UPGRADED LIFE

When you follow the 2-week plan closely, you're going to feel good—possibly better than you ever have before—and you can start making the best choices available so that becomes your new baseline. You have all of the information you need to feel that good all the time, or to figure out why you're not and take control to put yourself back in that state. This means not only performing at a higher level and sporting a hotter body, but also being stronger and more resilient than you ever imagined.

Most people forget they can feel this way, or they never get to experience it. They go their entire lives without ever knowing the level of focus you can achieve on this diet. They don't know the difference, but now you do, and that is a gift. You owe it to yourself to do something worthy of your time now that you have this increased energy and stamina. Don't waste your newfound power sitting on the couch or even checking out your new physique. (Okay, you can spend a few minutes each day doing that.) Instead, use it to do something meaningful, to change the world, or change your life for the better.

There's a reason I give so much information away for free on my Web site. It's because I spent so many years feeling sick and tired with a brain that wouldn't do what I wanted it to, and now I'm so grateful to be free of the weight and sluggishness that dragged me down. I don't want anyone else to have to go through what I did, and the more people I can share this information with, the happier I am. It's unfortunate that I had to spend so many years and so much money hacking myself to discover the Bulletproof Diet and why it works, but I did it so that you don't have to, and you can pay it forward by sharing this information with your friends and by using your Bulletproof mind and body to do something positive.

You just read an entire book about food, but the truth is that the Bulletproof Diet isn't really about food. The food you eat is merely a means to an end, and on the Bulletproof Diet, that end is being a better parent, a more creative artist, a more effective CEO, or a more energetic teacher. It's a way of turning on your human brain and allowing you to spend more time in a powerful state where stress isn't a factor and performance becomes effortless. I can't wait to hear about the amazing things you accomplish when you're Bulletproof. Now go out there and start kicking ass!

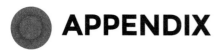

APPENDIX

BULLETPROOF RECIPES

Now that you know all the details of how the Bulletproof Diet is going to help you start looking great and kicking ass in all areas of life, it's time to start cooking some delicious kick-ass food. Here are some of my easiest, most impressive performance-boosting recipes. Of course, the quality of the results is somewhat dependent on the quality of ingredients you use. These recipes work better when you use the highest quality ingredients you can find, including organic, grass-fed animal products and organic produce. Do your best and enjoy!

BULLETPROOF COFFEE

Get ready to enjoy a high-performance buzz from your creamy mug of Bulletproof Coffee as you watch your chubby, tired coworkers eat low-fat yogurt and twigs for breakfast. It's almost unfair.

THE OFFICIAL BULLETPROOF COFFEE RECIPE

> 2 cups piping-hot brewed coffee made with Upgraded Coffee beans
>
> Up to 2 tablespoons grass-fed unsalted butter (use your hunger as a guide)
>
> Up to 2 tablespoons Brain Octane Oil (use your hunger as a guide)

BASIC BUTTER COFFEE RECIPE

> 2 cups piping-hot brewed coffee made with low-toxin beans
>
> Up to 2 tablespoons grass-fed unsalted butter (use your hunger as a guide)
>
> Up to 2 tablespoons coconut oil (use your hunger as a guide)

OPTIONAL ADD-INS:

Cinnamon (only the highest quality)

Vanilla powder

Chocolate powder

Stevia, erythritol, or hardwood xylitol to taste

Brew coffee as you normally would, but use a metal mesh filter if possible. A French press works well. As the coffee brews, pour hot tap water into your blender to preheat the blender. Empty the hot water from the blender when the coffee is ready. Add the brewed coffee, butter, and Brain Octane Oil into the blender. Close and cover the blender lid with a cloth in case the lid leaks. (You don't want hot coffee on the ceiling!) Blend until there's a thick layer of foam on top like a latte. Add cinnamon, vanilla, dark chocolate, or sweetener if desired.

> **TIP:** If you don't have a real blender, a hand blender (immersion blender) works okay but doesn't create as much foam as a high-powered blender.

NO-COFFEE VANILLA LATTE

This creamy hot beverage is the perfect replacement for coffee if you're pregnant or don't drink it for some other reason. Vanilla was originally used as a healing herb and has more antioxidants than almost any other food.

2 cups hot water

Up to 2 tablespoons grass-fed unsalted butter (use your hunger as a guide)

1 teaspoon vanilla powder

1 to 2 tablespoons coconut oil, Brain Octane Oil, or C8 MCT (use your hunger as a guide)

Stevia or hardwood xylitol to taste

Add all ingredients to a blender and blend until you have a creamy drink with a nice layer of foam on top. As with Bulletproof Coffee, an immersion blender works fine if you don't have a high-powered blender handy.

SMOKED SALMON AND AVOCADO "NOT-SUSHI"

This Bulletproof version of fast food takes only moments to prepare and provides plenty of healthy fats and proteins to keep you going for hours at warp speed. It's my go-to lunch when I'm in a rush and need something to sustain me.

1 Hass avocado

Cold smoked wild sockeye salmon

Sea salt

Cut the avocado into $1/2$-inch slices and the smoked salmon into strips. Wrap each slice of avocado in a piece of salmon and sprinkle with salt.

SMOKED SALMON BUTTER BITES

This is another Bulletproof fast food you can grab in a hurry. Try making this for lunch in your office kitchen and watch the look of confusion on your coworkers' faces as you start losing weight and looking great after eating butter for lunch!

Compound butter of your choice (see compound butter recipes on page 284)

Cold smoked wild salmon (look for Alaskan or sockeye salmon)

1 cucumber, cut into slices

Sea salt

Cut your compound butter into teaspoon-size pieces, roll a piece of salmon around each piece, and place the salmon-wrapped butter on top of a cucumber slice. Sprinkle with salt to taste and enjoy! This is like those cream cheese–salmon appetizer rolls, but without the inflammatory ingredients.

BULLETPROOF POACHED EGGS
WITH SAUTÉED GREENS

Poaching is a great Bulletproof method of cooking eggs to retain their nutrients and avoid damaging the proteins. This is a great weekend lunch meal that could easily be substituted for dinner. Try buying an assortment of fresh organic greens and prewash them when you get home so they're ready when you need them for easy cooking.

> 2 to 3 cups greens of your choice (kale, collards, chard, etc.)
>
> 2 tablespoons grass-fed unsalted butter or ghee
>
> Sea salt
>
> 2 tablespoons sliced raw cashews or almonds
>
> 2 poached eggs

Fill a pan with an inch or two of water and add the greens to cook. Once the greens are tender, drain the water and add the butter or ghee. Toss the greens in the butter or ghee until covered. Remove the greens from the heat and sprinkle with salt and nuts. You should poach your eggs so your yolks are runny and the nutrition from the yolks is intact. The restaurant tricks to poaching eggs are to add 2 tablespoons of apple cider vinegar to the water and then swirl the water around before cracking the eggs so they stay in the center of the whirlpool. Top your poached eggs with the greens.

BULLETPROOF TACO SALAD

When I make this, I like to prepare extra meat and save it for another meal or even eat it by itself for a quick lunch the next day. This satisfying meal can easily be eaten for dinner, too.

TACO MIX

1 pound grass-fed, organic fatty ground beef

2 tablespoons grass-fed unsalted butter or ghee

$\frac{1}{2}$ fresh lime, squeezed

1 to 2 tablespoons cayenne powder (warning: Suspect, don't use if you're sensitive!)

1 teaspoon dried oregano

Sea salt to taste

SALAD

1 cup spring lettuce

$\frac{1}{4}$ cup shredded red cabbage

2 shredded carrots

1 cucumber, cut into slices

$\frac{1}{2}$ avocado, sliced

"Creamy" Avocado Dressing (page 272)

To make the taco mix: In a medium pan, sauté the beef on medium-low until cooked gently but thoroughly. Your goal is not to brown the meat but to heat it enough that it's cooked through. Burned, caramelized meat tastes good, but it causes food cravings. Drain the excess liquid. Add the butter or ghee, lime juice, cayenne powder, oregano, and salt. Add more seasoning if you wish and play around with flavors!

To make the salad: Lay a bed with all of the salad ingredients, starting with the lettuce. Add a suitable portion of beef on top and then drizzle with dressing.

BULLETPROOF MEATBALLS

These meaty mouthfuls are great by themselves for lunch or for dinner with a vegetable side dish of your choice. Play around by adding chopped fresh herbs (basil, parsley, mint, oregano, sage, or rosemary) to see which you like best.

> 1 pastured whole egg
>
> $1/4$ cup ground almonds or almond butter
>
> Sea salt
>
> 1 tablespoon Brain Octane Oil
>
> 1 teaspoon ground turmeric
>
> 1 teaspoon chili powder
>
> 1 pound grass-fed, organic ground beef, bison, or lamb

Preheat the oven to 320°F.

Combine the egg, nuts, $1/2$ teaspoon salt, oil, turmeric, and chili powder and mix into the meat by hand to thoroughly combine. Form the meat into small balls the size of a Ping-Pong ball and place them on a rimmed baking sheet lined with foil. Sprinkle salt on the meatballs before placing them in the oven. Bake for 20 to 25 minutes, depending on the size of the meatball.

BULLETPROOF ONE-POT SOUP

This is a great way to use whatever veggies are in season at your local farmers' market or the ones that are sitting in your fridge. Make a big pot and bring it to work for lunch.

> 4 cups washed and loosely chopped Bulletproof vegetables of your choice (celery, fennel, cauliflower, broccoli, spinach, etc.)
>
> 8 cups filtered water or Upgraded Bone Broth (page 279)
>
> 1 cube (1 inch) fresh ginger, peeled and chopped
>
> Sea salt to taste
>
> Bouquet garni of fresh oregano and/or thyme
>
> 1 pound grass-fed, organic ground meat

Wash and chop your assortment of vegetables and boil it in the water or broth with the ginger, $1/2$ teaspoon salt, oregano, and thyme. Once the water comes to a boil, add the ground meat directly to the water. When the vegetables are tender and the meat is cooked thoroughly, remove from the heat, season with salt, and serve.

BULLETPROOF UN-OMELET

This is an amazing meal any time of day, but I like to eat it as a quick lunch. Once you're in maintenance mode, this is a great breakfast on days when you don't do Bulletproof Intermittent Fasting.

1 large head broccoli broken up into florets or 2 heads chopped fennel or 3 cups green beans (or any combination of these)

1 or 2 raw pastured egg yolks (duck if available)

1 tablespoon Brain Octane Oil

1 tablespoon lemon juice or apple cider vinegar

Fresh rosemary, oregano, or thyme

Sea salt

Steam the vegetables and drain well. In the meantime, pour hot tap water into your blender to preheat it. Empty the hot water from the blender when the vegetables are ready. Add $2/3$ of the vegetables, still piping hot, into the preheated blender along with the oil and vinegar. Immediately add the eggs. Allow the hot veggies to gently "cook" the eggs as you blend them on a low setting into a creamy sauce. Add the sauce back to the remaining vegetables. Sprinkle with herbs and salt to taste.

UPGRADED KALE SHAKE/SOUP

For this upgraded kale recipe, there is no need to add sugar, fruit, or any carbs for it to taste great and make you feel even better than a fruit/kale smoothie. Remember not to include the collagen or any other protein when eating this hot "shake" on protein fast days!

1 bunch dinosaur kale

500 milligrams calcium carbonate

Sea salt to taste

Herbs of choice (oregano rocks!)

1 to 4 teaspoons apple cider vinegar to taste

2 to 4 tablespoons grass-fed unsalted butter

1 to 2 tablespoons Brain Octane Oil

2 tablespoons high-quality, heat-stable protein (I recommend Upgraded Collagen)

Steam the kale with a cup or so of water until cooked (about 5 to 7 minutes). Drain the water. Add more fresh hot water if you want a thinner consistency. In a blender, combine the drained kale with the calcium carbonate, salt, herbs, vinegar, butter, and oil until super creamy. Last, for extra protein, add Upgraded Collagen or another heat-stable protein to the mixture and lightly blend until the protein is mixed in. Or just add pastured raw eggs!

> **Note:** Don't use this on your protein fast days and be sure to add the protein last and blend only slightly—you don't want to mechanically damage that expensive protein. You'll ruin it!

BULLETPROOF BENEDICT

Your favorite brunch is now Bulletproof.

    2 or 3 handfuls spinach, washed

    1 tablespoon grass-fed unsalted butter

    Sea salt to taste

    2 softly poached pastured eggs

    Bulletproof Hollandaise (recipe below)

    1 ripe avocado

In a pan, add the spinach with a tablespoon or two of water and sauté until just wilted. Drain the water and add the butter and a pinch of salt. Stir until the butter is melted and place the sautéed spinach on a plate. Place the poached eggs on the spinach and drizzle with hollandaise sauce. Halve and slice the avocado and place on a plate. Enjoy.

BULLETPROOF HOLLANDAISE

This delicious, creamy sauce is perfect on eggs but also satisfying on any protein or veggie of your choice.

    2 pastured egg yolks

    1 tablespoon lemon juice

    Pinch sea salt

    Dash cayenne powder (optional) (warning: Suspect, don't use if you're sensitive!)

    $\frac{1}{2}$ cup melted grass-fed unsalted butter or ghee

    Bunch fresh parsley (optional)

Place the egg yolks, lemon juice, salt, and cayenne pepper (if using) in a high-powered blender. Start the blender on low and run it for about 30 seconds. Slowly drizzle the melted butter or ghee into the blender. You must pour slowly to aid the emulsion. Once all the butter or ghee is added and the hollandaise has thickened, it's done. Top with parsley if you choose.

BULLETPROOF HASH

This quick hash is great for lunch or dinner on higher-carb days. For an extra boost, add cooked chopped spinach and/or half an avocado, diced, on top.

- 1 to 3 tablespoons pastured lard, bacon grease, or similar
- 1 small sweet potato, diced
- 1 teaspoon ground turmeric or grated turmeric root
- $\frac{1}{2}$ teaspoon sea salt
- $\frac{1}{2}$ teaspoon ground ginger or grated fresh ginger
- 1 to 2 tablespoons grass-fed unsalted butter or ghee
- 2 or 3 free-range eggs

In a skillet, heat the lard over medium heat and add the sweet potato, turmeric, salt, and ginger. Continue to cook until the sweet potato is soft. Melt the butter in another skillet over medium heat. In the second skillet, fry the eggs over easy or sunny side up. Serve the eggs on top of the hash and let the yolk drain into the hash.

ROASTED PORK BELLY WITH VEGETABLES

This recipe takes a little more time, but it's well worth it! Try making this for dinner on Sunday and eating the leftovers throughout the week. Make sure to use the highest-quality pork you can find, preferably from a local farmers' market. If you can't find good-quality pork, this recipe is great with any fatty grass-fed beef roast.

1 piece (1 to 2 pounds) pastured pork belly

2 tablespoons room-temperature grass-fed ghee, divided

3 or 4 carrots, peeled and cut into 2-inch pieces

3 celery stalks, cut into 2-inch pieces

1 fennel bulb, cut into $1/4$-inch slices

1 tablespoon chopped fresh thyme

1 tablespoon chopped fresh sage

1 tablespoon ground turmeric (optional)

Sea salt

$3/4$ cup water

1 tablespoon apple cider vinegar

2 tablespoons Brain Octane Oil

Preheat the oven to 320°F.

Score the pork skin and fat without cutting the meat. Rub 1 tablespoon of the ghee on the outside of the skin. In a roasting pan, lightly toss the carrots, celery, and fennel with the remaining ghee (it will melt anyway), thyme, sage, and turmeric (if using) and sprinkle with salt. Lay the pork belly meat side down in the pan on top of the vegetables and sprinkle the meat with salt.

Place the pork belly in the oven and roast for $1^1/_2$ hours. Combine the water and vinegar and pour the liquid into the pan. Roast for 1 more hour or until the meat pulls apart. After it's cooked, add the Brain Octane Oil to the vegetables.

OPTIONAL: Turn the oven to low broil for the last 10 minutes to create a crackling effect on the skin, but be careful not to char the meat.

BULLETPROOF ROAST WITH BRUSSELS SPROUTS

For this recipe you'll need a slow cooker, which is on the Suspect list because people tend to use it to overcook things. As long as you don't do that, it's a great tool that I recommend getting to make lots of Bulletproof dishes with minimal effort.

MEAT

    1 pound grass-fed, organic bottom sirloin or skirt steak

    2 tablespoons sea salt

    1 tablespoon ground turmeric

    1 teaspoon dried oregano

    2 tablespoons Brain Octane Oil

    3 tablespoons grass-fed unsalted butter

    $1\frac{1}{2}$ tablespoons apple cider vinegar

BRUSSELS SPROUTS

    1 pound Brussels sprouts (halved)

    2 tablespoons grass-fed unsalted butter

    2 teaspoons sea salt

    2 teaspoons ground turmeric

To make the meat: Coat the meat with the salt, turmeric, and oregano. Place the seasoned meat in the slow cooker and pour the Brain Octane Oil over the meat. Add the butter and slow cook on low for 6 to 8 hours or until the meat is shreddable. After the meat is cooked, add the vinegar.

    To make the Brussels sprouts: Preheat the oven to 300°F. Place the sprouts in a baking pan with the butter. Sprinkle on the salt and turmeric. Bake for 30 to 45 minutes.

BULLETPROOF STEW

This Bulletproof take on a classic, hearty dish will satisfy your body, mind, and soul.

Sea salt

1 to 2 pounds grass-fed, organic stewing beef (beef chuck), cut in 1-inch cubes

3 tablespoons ghee, divided

1 cube ($\frac{1}{2}$ inch) fresh ginger, peeled and thinly sliced

1 tablespoon ground turmeric

3 cups Upgraded Bone Broth (page 279) or 3 cups water + 3 tablespoons Upgraded Collagen

$\frac{1}{2}$ pound carrots, peeled and cut in 1-inch pieces

$\frac{1}{2}$ pound peeled and cubed sweet potatoes

1 large zucchini, cut in half moons

2 cups unsweetened coconut milk

1 tablespoon high-quality olive oil

Fresh cilantro, chopped

Lightly sprinkle salt on the meat cubes. Heat 1 to 2 tablespoons of the ghee in a pan on medium-high heat. When it starts to bubble slightly, brown all sides of the meat cubes in single-layer batches. Be careful not to burn the meat! The idea here is to seal in the juices but not cook the meat. Add the remaining ghee and the ginger and stir often until fragrant, about 2 minutes. Add the turmeric and stir frequently for 1 minute. Add the broth or water with collagen and the beef and bring to a boil, stirring the sides and bottom of the pan to ensure nothing is stuck to the bottom. Reduce the heat to medium-low, cover, and simmer, stirring occasionally, for 45 minutes to 1 hour or until the meat is tender. Add the carrots and sweet potatoes and simmer for 15 minutes. Add the zucchini and simmer for 5 to 10 more minutes. Stir in the coconut milk and olive oil. Garnish with cilantro and serve.

ROASTED LAMB RACK WITH VEGETABLES

Grass-fed lamb is one of the most Bulletproof proteins on the planet, and it shines here in this simple, classic preparation.

1 tablespoon ghee

1 American rack of grass-fed, organic lamb (8 chops)
or 2 New Zealand racks of grass-fed, organic lamb (16 chops total), about 1½ pounds

1 tablespoon each fresh chopped sage, thyme, oregano, rosemary, and ground turmeric, to taste

Sea salt

2 cups sliced fennel

2 cups sliced celery

2 cups sliced cauliflower

Preheat the oven to 350°F.

Rub the ghee into the rack. Score the fat on the top diagonally. Add the chopped herbs and the salt. Place the vegetables in the pan and lay the lamb fat side up in a roasting pan on top of the bed of vegetables. Bake until a thermometer inserted into the lamb registers 125° to 130°F, about 45 minutes. Turn the oven to low broil for a few minutes at the end to crisp the skin. Avoid overbrowning or charring.

BP PULLED SOMETHING!

This is another recipe that requires a slow cooker—and once you taste it, you'll be so glad you have one! Use pastured pork shoulder if you can find it from a good source or grass-fed beef roast.

> 6 strips uncooked, high-quality pastured bacon
>
> 4 pounds pastured pork shoulder or grass-fed, organic beef roast
>
> Sea salt to taste
>
> 2 tablespoons dried oregano
>
> 1 tablespoon ground turmeric

Place the bacon strips at the base of the slow cooker. Salt the roast, rub in the oregano and turmeric, and add it to the slow cooker. Cook on low for 14 to 16 hours, depending on desired crispiness. Shred the meat with a fork. You can eat this plain, but if you want to add an amazing, tangy sweet-and-sour barbecue flavor, combine the juice from the meat with about $1/2$ cup each of xylitol and apple cider vinegar and use it as a sauce.

OVEN BURGERS

Meat on meat—need I say more?

> 2 pounds grass-fed, organic beef or lamb
>
> 2 tablespoons dried oregano
>
> 1 tablespoon dried rosemary
>
> 2 teaspoons ground turmeric
>
> Sea salt
>
> 4 large slices pastured, preservative-free bacon

Preheat the oven to 325°F.

Form the meat into 8 burgers. Rub the herbs and salt on the meat directly. Place $1/2$ strip of bacon on each burger. Bake for 15 to 20 minutes or until the bacon is golden on the outside and the burger is cooked thoroughly.

BULLETPROOF BAKED FISH

This "fish rub" can be used on pork or beef, but I especially like it with a nice piece of wild-caught baked fish.

$\frac{1}{4}$ cup ground coffee beans

$\frac{1}{4}$ teaspoon vanilla powder

Hardwood xylitol to taste (about 3 tablespoons)

1 tablespoon ground turmeric

1 tablespoon dried oregano

2 tablespoons sea salt

1 pound tilapia, trout, or other Bulletproof protein of your choice

Combine the ingredients for the seasoning and rub generously onto the fish. Bake at 320°F until cooked through.

CAULIFLOWER-BACON MASH

You will never miss eating mashed potatoes when you can have this delicious creamy, bacon-flavored mashed cauliflower instead!

1 large head cauliflower, cut into florets

4 tablespoons grass-fed unsalted butter

2 tablespoons Brain Octane Oil

$\frac{1}{2}$ tablespoon apple cider vinegar

Sea salt to taste

$\frac{1}{2}$ pound pastured, preservative-free bacon lightly cooked at medium-low (not crispy—keep those fats intact), diced

Steam the cauliflower until tender, drain, and blend $\frac{3}{4}$ of the cauliflower with all other ingredients except the bacon in a high-powered blender. Stir in the bacon. Pulse until chunky. For amazing flavor, add 1 to 2 tablespoons of the bacon grease (as long as it didn't smoke when you were cooking it at a low temperature).

"CHEESY" BUTTERNUT SQUASH

This is a great side dish that you can even eat in larger quantities as a main dish on your higher-carb days. The creaminess gives it a cheeselike consistency with no dairy!

1 medium butternut squash, seeded and cut into 1-inch cubes

3 or 4 medium carrots, peeled and cut into 1-inch pieces

4 tablespoons grass-fed unsalted butter

$\frac{1}{2}$ tablespoon apple cider vinegar

1 spring onion, cut into 4 pieces

2 to 3 tablespoons Brain Octane Oil

Sea salt to taste

Steam the squash and carrots until tender and then drain thoroughly. Make sure to remove as much water as possible. Add the cooked squash and carrots to the blender along with the remaining ingredients and blend until smooth.

CREAMED VEGETABLES

The butter and method used here will give the veggies a creamy consistency without using any cream. Try the same method with any other Bulletproof vegetables of your choice.

1 bunch asparagus, broccoli, and/or green beans

3 tablespoons grass-fed unsalted butter

2 tablespoons Brain Octane Oil

$\frac{1}{2}$ tablespoon apple cider vinegar

Bunch fresh herbs of your choice (parsley, cilantro, oregano, dill, sage, and/or thyme)

Sea salt to taste

Steam the veggies until just tender. Remove $\frac{1}{3}$ of the vegetables while hot and put them in the blender. Add the rest of the ingredients (except the remaining veggies) and blend until smooth and creamy. Drizzle this mixture over the remaining vegetables.

BAKED BROCCOLI WITH TURMERIC + GINGER

The turmeric and ginger give this side dish an extra anti-inflammatory boost! Try eating a big bowl of this for lunch or dinner after eating some nutritional Kryptonite at your last meal.

$1/2$ tablespoon grass-fed unsalted butter or ghee

1 stalk lemongrass

1 chunk (1 inch) fresh ginger, peeled and minced

1 tablespoon ground turmeric

2 tablespoons Brain Octane Oil

1 head broccoli, cut into florets

Sea salt to taste

Preheat the oven to 320°F.

Add the butter or ghee, lemongrass, and ginger to a medium pot. Turn the heat on low and stir often for 20 to 30 minutes until the flavors have infused. Make sure it does not boil! Once infused, add the turmeric and stir. Rub the oil onto the broccoli florets, sprinkle with salt, and put into the oven. Bake for 30 minutes, stirring every 10 minutes. Strain the contents of the pot and drizzle or toss through the broccoli. Sprinkle with salt to taste.

LIME-CILANTRO CAULIFLOWER "NOT-RICE"

It can be a little tricky to get the right texture here, so play around with a grater and/or a food processor until the cauliflower is roughly the size and shape of rice. This is a great side dish with a surprising amount of flavor that goes nicely with fish or meat.

1 head cauliflower

2 tablespoons grass-fed unsalted butter

Juice from 1 whole lime

2 tablespoons Brain Octane Oil

$1/2$ cup chopped fresh cilantro

Sea salt to taste

1 spring onion, chopped (optional)

Grate the cauliflower or use a food processor to pulse it into the right texture.

Heat a large sauté pan to medium and melt the butter. When the butter is melted, add the riced cauliflower. Don't be afraid to crowd the pan, as it will aid in the cooking process by creating a steamer effect. *Caution:* You don't want to brown the cauliflower. Cook it gently for 5 to 10 minutes, stirring and turning over often. Once the cauliflower is cooked through, turn off the heat and add the lime juice, oil, cilantro, and salt to taste. Mix evenly in the pan and transfer to a dish for serving. Garnish with spring onion (if using).

BULLETPROOF SWEET POTATO–GINGER SOUP

This satisfying soup makes a great lunch or dinner on your protein fast days. While this recipe creates a smooth, silky soup, you can customize it by skipping the final step in the blender if you prefer a chunky texture.

2 tablespoons Brain Octane Oil

3 cups (1/2-inch) cubed, peeled sweet potatoes

1 1/2 cups (1/4-inch) sliced, peeled carrots

1 tablespoon freshly grated ginger

3 cups water

1/2 teaspoon sea salt

2 tablespoons grass-fed unsalted butter

Heat the oil in a large saucepan over medium-low heat. Add the sweet potatoes, carrots, and ginger and cook for 2 minutes. Add the water, cover, and simmer for 30 minutes or until the vegetables are tender. Stir in the salt. Pour into a blender or food processor or use a hand mixer to blend until smooth. Add the butter and blend again.

UPGRADED ICEBERG SALAD

While iceberg lettuce is lower in nutrients than other types of lettuce, it's also lower in protein. Since you'll be eating this on protein fast days, iceberg is the best choice. You can add other vegetables to this salad. Just be careful, because some vegetables have more protein than others. These were chosen specifically because they are low in protein.

1 head iceberg lettuce, chopped

1 small bunch radishes, thinly sliced

$\frac{1}{2}$ avocado, sliced

$\frac{1}{2}$ cup olives, pitted and chopped

$\frac{1}{2}$ cucumber, thinly sliced

Add as many or as few of these ingredients as you like and top with the Bulletproof salad dressing of your choice (see recipes that follow).

BULLETPROOF SALAD DRESSINGS

For all of the dressings below, combine all ingredients in a blender and blend until smooth and creamy. Try them on salads, cooked vegetables, and even baked sweet potatoes.

"CREAMY" AVOCADO DRESSING

$\frac{1}{2}$ avocado

1 to 2 tablespoons Brain Octane Oil

1 tablespoon apple cider vinegar

1 tablespoon fresh lemon juice

1 cup sliced cucumber

$\frac{1}{4}$ cup chopped fresh cilantro

1 spring onion (optional)

Sea salt to taste

BULLETPROOF HONEY-MUSTARD VINAIGRETTE

$\frac{1}{4}$ cup apple cider vinegar

$\frac{1}{8}$ cup extra virgin olive oil

$\frac{1}{8}$ cup Brain Octane Oil

1 tablespoon mustard

2 tablespoons raw honey (or hardwood xylitol)

BULLETPROOF CREAMY BASIL VINAIGRETTE

$\frac{1}{2}$ avocado

$\frac{1}{4}$ cup extra virgin olive oil

2 tablespoons Brain Octane Oil

$\frac{1}{4}$ cup apple cider vinegar

Small handful fresh basil leaves

BULLETPROOF RANCH DRESSING

1 cup Bulletproof Mayonnaise (page 274)

2 tablespoons chopped fresh dill

1 tablespoon apple cider vinegar

2 cloves garlic, minced together with sea salt

Sea salt to taste

Chill for a few hours after blending.

BAKED CARROT FRIES

These make a great side dish for any meal on protein fast days or with dinner anytime you like.

    6 to 8 medium carrots, peeled and cut into sticks

    3 to 4 tablespoons grass-fed unsalted butter or compound butter of your choice

    Sea salt to taste

Preheat the oven to 320°F. Lay the carrot sticks on a baking sheet and bake until they reach the desired tenderness. Remove from the oven, toss with butter, and sprinkle with salt. On days you are not doing Bulletproof Protein Fasting, enjoy these with Bulletproof Mayonnaise (recipe below)!

BULLETPROOF MAYONNAISE

This is delicious with Baked Carrot Fries, on top of sweet potatoes, or along with any protein you like. If your mayo won't emulsify, try adding a chunk of avocado, another egg yolk, or some soy lecithin. I like to add fresh herbs to flavor my mayo, too! Unfortunately, this has too much protein for protein fast days.

    1 large egg

    $^3/_4$ cup extra light olive oil

    $^1/_4$ cup Brain Octane Oil

    2 to 3 teaspoons lemon or lime juice (fresh squeezed)

    Pinch sea salt

Add all of the ingredients together in a bowl and let the egg sink to the bottom. Using an immersion blender, combine all of the ingredients until the mayo reaches the desired consistency. This recipe yields about $1^1/_2$ cups of mayo. If your mayo is not gelling, just add $^1/_2$ avocado and it will be amazing.

BULLETPROOF BEAN-FREE DAHL AND RICE

This is a delicious vegetarian meal option for protein fast days or whenever you can't get your hands on some grass-fed meat.

2 cups basmati white rice

4 medium carrots

1 beet

1 cup (or 5 leaves) rainbow chard

2 cups (or 1 large floret) broccoli (without the stems)

2 thin slices fresh turmeric root

2 thin slices fresh ginger

4 tablespoons grass-fed unsalted butter or ghee

2 tablespoons Brain Octane Oil

$\frac{1}{2}$ teaspoon apple cider vinegar

Sea salt

Cayenne powder (warning: Suspect, don't use if you're sensitive!)

Fresh washed cilantro, chopped

Rinse the rice 5 or 6 times. Keep rinsing it in tap water until the frothy white suds and particles are gone. Drain the tap water and then fill the pan back up with the correct amount of filtered water for the amount of rice you are cooking. Put your rice on the stove (or in your rice cooker) on medium and begin cooking.

Wash the carrots, beet, chard, and broccoli thoroughly and cut into 1-inch pieces. If you have a high-powered blender, you can leave the vegetable chunks fairly large, but if you have a smaller blender, it helps to cut them up closer to a dice. Steam the vegetables, turmeric, and ginger with filtered water for 7 to 10 minutes. You want your vegetables to be firm but soft enough to poke with a fork. Overcooking them diminishes the nutrients. Put all the vegetables into a blender and add the butter or ghee, oil, vinegar, and $\frac{1}{2}$ teaspoon salt. Blend for 1 to 2 minutes until smooth.

Fill each bowl halfway with rice and top the bowl with a large ladle of your vegetable soup. Add a sprinkle of cayenne powder on top. Add salt to taste. Sprinkle with cilantro to garnish.

BULLETPROOF CARROT-FENNEL SOUP WITH RICE

This is a light, delicious soup that's perfect for protein fast days. If you like, add white rice to the soup and eat it as a satisfying dinner. Play around with the texture, making this as smooth or as chunky as you like.

    2 celery stalks

    2 pounds carrots

    2 medium fennel bulbs

    2 tablespoons Brain Octane Oil

    1 chunk (2 inches) fresh ginger, peeled and finely chopped

    2 tablespoons grass-fed unsalted butter

    1 cup cooked white rice (optional)

Finely chop the celery and cut the carrots and fennel into 1-inch chunks. Heat the oil in a soup pot over medium heat. Add the celery, carrots, fennel, and ginger and cook until all ingredients are mixed and softened. Add 4 cups of water, mix well, cover, and cook for 40 minutes to 1 hour over medium heat. Blend well using an immersion blender or traditional blender. Add the butter and then blend again. If desired, fill the bowl halfway with cooked white rice before adding the soup.

LEMON RICE

This simple and delicious version of white rice is the perfect side dish to eat on protein fast days or alongside a nice piece of Bulletproof meat once or twice a week for dinner.

    4 tablespoons ($\frac{1}{2}$ stick) grass-fed unsalted butter or ghee, divided

    2 to 3 cups cooked white rice

    Sea salt to taste

    Freshly squeezed juice of 2 lemons, plus more if needed

    1 to 2 tablespoons Brain Octane Oil

    1 lemon, quartered

Heat half of the butter or ghee in a saucepot over medium-low heat. Spoon in the cooked rice and stir. Add salt to taste and then add $\frac{3}{4}$ of the lemon juice. Cook for 1 to 5 minutes, stirring frequently, until hot. Stir in the remaining butter and cook for 1 more minute. Place the rice on a platter and sprinkle on the rest of the lemon juice and the oil. Use the lemon quarters to make your plates look fancy!

BAKED SWEET POTATOES

Think of this as a palette for you to turn into your masterpiece by playing around with various Bulletproof toppings. Instead of bacon, feel free to add avocado slices, Bulletproof Mayonnaise (page 274), veggies, ground meat, or just more butter!

3 or 4 medium sweet potatoes

3 to 4 tablespoons grass-fed unsalted butter or Bulletproof compound butter of your choice

3 to 4 tablespoons chopped bacon (optional)

Sea salt to taste

Preheat the oven to 320°F. Wash and dry the sweet potatoes. Line a rimmed baking sheet with foil and use a fork to prick holes on all sides of the potatoes. Bake them for 50 to 60 minutes, depending on size. Test with a fork and remove from the oven when done. Cut a lengthwise slit in the top and pinch the sides. Add your desired amount of butter, bacon (if using), and salt.

UPGRADED GUACAMOLE

This is one of my favorite recipes—delicious, creamy guacamole with an extra brain boost from Brain Octane Oil that keeps you full longer than regular guacamole. eat it with cucumber or celery sticks for lunch or on top of a protein of your choice for dinner! I've been known to just eat a bowl of it with a spoon.

> 4 large, ripe Hass avocados, peeled
>
> 2 to 4 tablespoons Brain Octane Oil (note: coconut oil is not a good substitute here, since the flavor does not go well with avocados)
>
> 2 teaspoons or more sea salt (to taste)
>
> 1 tablespoon dried oregano
>
> 1 to 3 teaspoons apple cider vinegar or lime (to taste)
>
> Pinch of ascorbic acid, aka vitamin C powder (optional, prevents browning)

Blend everything with a hand blender until it's very creamy. Stir in chopped cilantro or other herbs of your choice.

BULLETPROOF CHICKEN BREAST

Chicken is an inferior source of protein and fat compared to lamb, beef, or fish, and most of it is poorly fed with GMO feed, antibiotics, and poorly stored grains that add toxins to the meat. But it's cheap, and some people actually like it! Try this recipe once you're in maintenance mode and track your body's response.

> 2 grass-fed, organic bone-in chicken breasts, skin removed
>
> Juice of 1 lemon
>
> 1 teaspoon dry mustard powder
>
> $\frac{1}{4}$ cup each chopped fresh basil, thyme, and oregano
>
> Sea salt to taste
>
> 2 tablespoons ghee

Wash and dry the chicken breasts and set aside. Combine the lemon juice, dry mustard, herbs, and salt. In a baking dish, drizzle the lemon juice mixture over the chicken breast and place back in the fridge for 1 hour, rotating after 30 minutes. Place 1 tablespoon ghee on top of each breast. Preheat the oven to 320°F. Bake the chicken for 45 minutes or until cooked through.

UPGRADED BONE BROTH

This broth is great to use in soup recipes, and those hard-core folks can even try drinking it for a high-performance shot of healthy animal fat!

3 medium carrots, peeled and cut into rough chunks

3 stalks celery, peeled and cut into rough chunks

2½ pounds assorted beef marrow bones

1 fresh bouquet garni (your choice of fresh oregano, rosemary, thyme, sage, etc.)

1 to 2 tablespoons apple cider vinegar

1 cup Upgraded Collagen per liter of broth (optional)

Sea salt to taste

In a large stockpot, lightly sauté the carrots and celery for a few minutes until translucent. Add the beef bones and bouquet garni and cover with water. Add the apple cider vinegar to the water, as it helps draw out the nutrients from the bones. Simmer on a low heat (do not boil) for anywhere between 8 and 14 hours. After your broth has reached the desired color and flavor, remove the bones and strain the vegetables out. Add the appropriate amount of collagen (if using) for the amount of broth and stir until dissolved. Optional: Add salt to taste at this point and then store in mason jars for future use.

SHOCKINGLY RICH CHOCOLATE TRUFFLE PUDDING

When you use the best-quality ingredients, desserts like this are nutrient-rich foods that will help you lose weight instead of Kryptonite that will leave you inflamed and craving more. *Tip:* Use Grass-Fed Bulletproof CollaGelatin to provide 2 times the protein of normal gelatin.

   4 cups full-fat coconut milk, BPA-free, divided

   Up to 4 tablespoons hardwood xylitol or stevia (to taste)

   1 tablespoon grass-fed gelatin (or 2 tablespoons Grass-Fed Bulletproof CollaGelatin)

   2 teaspoons vanilla powder

   $3/4$ cup chocolate powder

   4 tablespoons grass-fed unsalted butter

   1 tablespoon coconut oil or Brain Octane Oil

   $1/4$ cup macadamia nuts plus additional for topping (optional)

Heat 1 cup of the coconut milk, the xylitol, and the gelatin in a saucepan over medium heat until dissolved. Place the remaining 3 cups of coconut milk in a blender with the vanilla, chocolate powder, butter, and oil. Blend thoroughly. Add the hot coconut milk/gelatin mixture to the blender and pulse until mixed, with or without the macadamia nuts. Pour the entire blender contents into muffin tins or ramekins and place in the fridge for an hour to set. Top with more nuts (if using).

ALMOND TRUFFLE CUPS

This takes the truffle pudding (above) to a whole new level with the addition of almond butter and even more butter!

   1 recipe Shockingly Rich Chocolate Truffle Pudding

   $1/2$ cup raw almond butter

   2 tablespoons grass-fed unsalted butter

   2 tablespoons hardwood xylitol or stevia to taste

   Dash sea salt

Prepare the pudding. Before pouring the contents into muffin tins or ramekins, mix the almond butter, butter, xylitol, and salt together. Line the muffin cups with a layer of the almond butter mixture. Pour the pudding on top and let it set in the fridge for an hour.

COCONUT-BLUEBERRY ULTIMATELY CREAMY PANNA COTTA

One of the best parts of the Bulletproof Diet is being able to eat delectable desserts like this on a regular basis. *Tip:* Use Grass-Fed Bulletproof CollaGelatin to provide twice the protein of normal gelatin.

1 cup fresh or frozen blueberries

4 cups full-fat coconut milk, BPA-free, divided

Up to 4 tablespoons hardwood xylitol or stevia (to taste)

1 tablespoon grass-fed gelatin (or 2 tablespoons Grass-Fed Bulletproof CollaGelatin)

2 teaspoons vanilla powder

4 tablespoons grass-fed unsalted butter

1 tablespoon coconut oil or Brain Octane Oil

$\frac{1}{2}$ cup shredded coconut

Place the berries in a deep-sided dish. Heat 1 cup of the coconut milk, the xylitol, and the gelatin in a saucepan over medium heat until dissolved. Place the remaining 3 cups of coconut milk in a blender with the vanilla, butter, and oil. Blend thoroughly and then add the hot coconut milk/gelatin mixture and shredded coconut. Pulse the blender until mixed. Pour the entire blender contents over the blueberries and place the dish in the fridge for an hour to set. Add more berries to the top!

CREAMY COCONUT "GET SOME" ICE CREAM

This Paleo-friendly ice cream proves once and for all that ice cream doesn't have to be a "cheat" food. With this recipe, ice cream is now a health food.

4 whole pastured eggs

4 pastured egg yolks (in addition to the whole eggs above)

2 teaspoons vanilla powder

1 gram vitamin C (ascorbic acid) or 10 drops apple cider vinegar or lime juice to taste

7 tablespoons grass-fed unsalted butter

7 tablespoons coconut oil

3 tablespoons + 2 teaspoons Brain Octane Oil

$5\frac{1}{2}$ tablespoons hardwood xylitol or erythritol (or more to taste—you can add up to 160 grams if you want)

$\frac{1}{4}$ to $\frac{1}{2}$ cup chocolate powder (optional)

About $\frac{1}{2}$ cup water or ice (use less than you think you need, then increase the amount if necessary)

Blend all ingredients except the water or ice in a blender until soft and creamy. Add water or ice and blend some more until well blended. Ideally, you want a yogurtlike consistency for creamy ice cream, or add more water for a firmer, icier texture. Pour the mixture into an ice cream maker and turn it on. This will make perfect-consistency ice cream. Enjoy!

BULLETPROOF CUPCAKES

It took me many years, but I finally figured out how to make baked goods Bulletproof. This will soon be one of your favorite foods on the Bulletproof Diet!

12 tablespoons erythritol or hardwood xylitol or a 50/50 mix (best)

12 ounces 85% or darker chocolate, chopped or chips

$^3/_4$ cup grass-fed unsalted butter, at room temperature

Tiny pinch sea salt

6 eggs at room temperature, separated

2+ teaspoons vanilla extract or 1 teaspoon ground vanilla

1 teaspoon cocoa powder (or very finely ground coffee beans)

1 tablespoon sweet rice flour (omit if you can't find it and do NOT use normal rice flour, which is gritty)

Preheat the oven to 350°F.

Line 18 muffin tin cups with paper liners. If you'd like to make a dozen, reduce the recipe by $^1/_3$. If you'd like to make 2 dozen, increase the recipe by $^1/_3$. Powder the erythritol and/or xylitol in a blender. Make sure to pulse it so friction doesn't melt the xylitol into a sticky mess! Set aside. Melt the chocolate and butter in a heavy, medium saucepan over low heat, stirring constantly, until smooth. Remove from the heat and stir often as it cools a little. Set aside. Mix 6 tablespoons of the powdered xylitol/erythritol, salt, and all 6 egg yolks and beat on medium to high speed for about 3 minutes until you get something very thick and pale. Using a spatula, fold the egg-xylitol blend into the still-warm chocolate and add the vanilla, cocoa powder or coffee, and flour. Use a separate bowl to beat the egg whites on high speed until soft peaks form. Then slowly add the remaining 6 tablespoons of xylitol/erythritol and beat until medium-firm peaks form. Fold the egg whites into the chocolate–egg yolk mixture little by little, in 3 or 4 batches.

Fill the cupcake liners $^3/_4$ full and bake for 11 minutes. Rotate the pan and bake for 11 more minutes. Use a wire rack to let them cool completely. If you want to make a frosting, use the sweetener of your choice mixed with grass-fed butter, cocoa powder, and vanilla.

BULLETPROOF BERRY BOWL

This simple combination of low-sugar fruits will give you an easy, delicious dessert for any day of the week.

$1/2$ cup blueberries

$1/2$ cup raspberries

$1/2$ cup strawberries, stems removed and chopped

Juice of $1/2$ lemon

$1/4$ cup chopped fresh basil

Combine the berries, squeeze the lemon juice over the fruit, and stir. Top with chopped basil for an elegant touch.

BULLETPROOF COMPOUND BUTTERS

Compound butters are great on meat and vegetables or when used in cooking to add more satisfying healthy fat to any hot dish. You can also use them as an amazing spread on gluten-free Mary's Gone Crackers to create a quick lunch that satisfies for hours. You can make compound butters and freeze them for later, which is a great way to preserve fresh herbs. For each compound butter recipe, allow the butter to reach room temperature and blend all ingredients together. Add salt to taste.

SAVORY COMPOUND BUTTER

1 cup grass-fed unsalted butter

3 to 4 tablespoons chopped fresh herbs of your choice (parsley, cilantro, oregano, dill, sage, rosemary, thyme, etc.)

Sea salt to taste

BERRY COMPOUND BUTTER

1 cup grass-fed unsalted butter

$1/4$ cup fresh berries (blackberries, strawberries, or blueberries)

Dash cinnamon (only the highest quality)

Hardwood xylitol or raw honey to taste for sweetness

Dash sea salt

COCOA COMPOUND BUTTER

1 cup grass-fed unsalted butter

3 tablespoons raw cocoa

Dash cinnamon (only the highest quality)

Hardwood xylitol, stevia, or dash of raw honey to taste for sweetness

Dash sea salt

GHEE

It's actually quite easy to make your own ghee at home. The amount of ghee you get from a pound of butter actually depends on what quality butter you use, because cheap butter contains a lot of water and some chemicals. Good-quality butter is 84 percent fat, so you'll get about $1\frac{1}{2}$ cups of ghee from a pound of butter as long as you use the highest-quality grass-fed butter every time!

1 pound grass-fed butter

In a pot, melt the butter on low heat and let the milk solids bubble to the surface. Skim those bubbles until there is just a layer of protein at the bottom of the pan. Let it brown slightly but be careful not to let it burn! Strain the contents of the pan over a mesh strainer covered with cheesecloth into a clean jar.

NOTES

Chapter 1

1   Aggarwal BB, Shishodia S, Sandur SK, Pandey MK, and Sethi G. Inflammation and cancer: How hot is the link? *Biochemical Pharmacology* 2006;72(11):1605–1621.

2   Giugliano D, Ceriello A, Esposito K. The effects of diet on inflammation: Emphasis on the metabolic syndrome. *Journal of the American College of Cardiology* 2006;48(4):677–685.

3   Zhang J. Yin and yang interplay of IFN-gamma in inflammation and autoimmune disease. Journal of *Clinical Investigation* 2007;117(4):871–873. www.medscape.com/viewarticle/776988

4   www.springerlink.com/content/la19dubvrja6l84v

5   www.biomedcentral.com/1472-6823/5/10

6   www.ncbi.nlm.nih.gov/pubmed/10395614

7   www.ncbi.nlm.nih.gov/pubmed/14726276

8   www.ncbi.nlm.nih.gov/pubmed/7759018

9   www.springerlink.com/content/43254u3310042577

10 www.ncbi.nlm.nih.gov/pubmed/16129731

11 www.ncbi.nlm.nih.gov/pubmed/15111494

12 www.ncbi.nlm.nih.gov/pubmed/9316457

13 www.ncbi.nlm.nih.gov/pubmed/20150284

14 www.ncbi.nlm.nih.gov/pubmed/22289055

15 www.ncbi.nlm.nih.gov/pubmed/20566347

16 www.ncbi.nlm.nih.gov/pubmed/11192627

17 www.sciencedirect.com/science/article/pii/S096399699600066X

18 www.sciencemag.org/content/328/5975/228.abstract

19 www.nature.com/nature/journal/v444/n7122/abs/4441022a.html

20 www.ncbi.nlm.nih.gov/pubmed/21587065

Chapter 2 Endnotes

1   www.nytimes.com/2011/08/21/magazine/do-you-suffer-from-decision-fatigue.html

2   www.nytimes.com/2007/10/09/science/09tier.

3   www.ncbi.nlm.nih.gov/pmc/articles/PMC2673878

4   www.ncbi.nlm.nih.gov/pubmed/16366738

5   www.ncbi.nlm.nih.gov/pubmed/18395289

6   www.fasebj.org/cgi/content/meeting_abstract/27/1_MeetingAbstracts/951.1

7   www.jnutbio.com/article/S0955-2863(14)00020-5/abstract

8   www.ncbi.nlm.nih.gov/pmc/articles/PMC3153489

9   http://ajh.oxfordjournals.org/content/25/7/727.short

10 www.ncbi.nlm.nih.gov/pubmed/18640459; http://onlinelibrary.wiley.com/doi/10.1111/j.1365-2362.2012.02719.x/abstract

11 www.mayomedicallaboratories.com/test-catalog/Clinical+and+Interpretive/80308

12 Alice Feinstein, ed. *Prevention's Healing with Vitamins*. Emmaus, PA: Rodale, 1996.

Chapter 3

1   http://annals.org/article.aspx?articleid=1846638

2   www.jissn.com/content/3/2/12

3   www.ncbi.nlm.nih.gov/pubmed/16500874

4   www.ncbi.nlm.nih.gov/pubmed/18641180

5   www.ncbi.nlm.nih.gov/pubmed/7096916

6   Bird AR, Brown IL, Topping DL. Starch, resistant starch, the gut microflora and human health. *Current Issues in Intestinal Microbiology.* 2000;1:25-37.
7   www.sciencedirect.com/science/article/pii/S0306452210012947
8   www.nature.com/ejcn/journal/v62/n4/abs/1602866a.html
9   www.allergykids.com/index.php?id=4
10   aje.oxfordjournals.org/content/147/4/342.short
      ajpheart.physiology.org/content/293/5/H2919
      www.ncbi.nlm.nih.gov/pubmed/17854706
      www.karger.com/Article/Abstract/73797
      www.ncbi.nlm.nih.gov/pubmed/18636564
11   www.ncbi.nlm.nih.gov/pubmed/9872614
12   www.ncbi.nlm.nih.gov/pubmed/6299329
13   www.ncbi.nlm.nih.gov/pubmed/17003019
14   http://onlinelibrary.wiley.com/doi/10.1002/oby.20501/abstract
15   www.ncbi.nlm.nih.gov/pubmed/11024006
16   http://onlinelibrary.wiley.com/doi/10.1002/oby.20501/abstract
17   www.ncbi.nlm.nih.gov/pubmed/21094734
18   L.J. Harris. *Vitamins in Theory and Practice.* New York: Macmillan, 1935, p. 224.
19   www.specialnutrients.com/pdf/book/Mycotoxins%20and%20mycotoxicosis%20in%20humans%20 and%20animals%20Book%20Gimeno%20security.pdf, p. 70.
20   www.ncbi.nlm.nih.gov/pubmed/3265709
21   www.sciencedirect.com/science/article/pii/S1053811906006902

Chapter 4

1   http://rsna2005.rsna.org/rsna2005/V2005/conference/event_display.cfm?em_id=4418422
2   http://news.aces.illinois.edu/content/caffeine-may-block-inflammation-linked-mild-cognitive-impairment
3   www.ncbi.nlm.nih.gov/pubmed/21046357
4   www.nutritionj.com/content/pdf/1475-2891-10-61.pdf
5   www.ncbi.nlm.nih.gov/pubmed/21037214
6   http://well.blogs.nytimes.com/2011/09/26/coffee-drinking-linked-to-less-depression-in-women
7   www.ncbi.nlm.nih.gov/pubmed/21949167
8   www.mendeley.com/research/protective-effects-kahweol-cafestol-against-hydrogen-peroxideinduced-oxidative-stress-dna-damage
9   www.mendeley.com/catalog/cafestol-extraction-yield-different-coffee-brew-mechanisms
10   http://microbewiki.kenyon.edu/index.php/Gut_Microbiota_and_Obesity
11   www.ncbi.nlm.nih.gov/pmc/articles/PMC524219
12   www.jnutbio.com/article/S0955-2863%2814%2900020-5/abstract?elsca1=etoc&elsca2=email&elsca3 =0955-2863_201404_25_4&elsca4=nutrition_dietetics
13   www.ncbi.nlm.nih.gov/pubmed/21627318
14   www.mdpi.com/2072-6643/3/10/858
15   www.mendeley.com/catalog/stimulation-mild-sustained-ketonemia-mediumchain-triacylglycerols-healthy-humans-estimated-potential
16   *Eat, Fast, and Live Longer.* Episode 3, "Horizon." BBC, 2012–2013. www.bbc.co.uk/programmes/ b01lxyzc. [television series]
17   www.ncbi.nlm.nih.gov/pubmed/12558961
18   www.ncbi.nlm.nih.gov/pubmed/23512957
19   www.ncbi.nlm.nih.gov/pmc/articles/PMC524219
20   www.ncbi.nlm.nih.gov/pubmed/19945408

Chapter 5

1   http://health.ucsd.edu/news/2002/02_08_Kripke.html
2   www.ncbi.nlm.nih.gov/pubmed/12123620
3   www.ncbi.nlm.nih.gov/pubmed/14737168
4   www.ncbi.nlm.nih.gov/pubmed/11511309
5   www.webmd.com/sleep-disorders/excessive-sleepiness-10/diabetes-lack-of-sleep

6   www.ncbi.nlm.nih.gov/pubmed/20051441
7   www.medicalnewstoday.com/releases/74081.php
8   www.alzforum.org/news/research-news/brain-drain-glymphatic-pathway-clears-av-requires-water-channel
9   www.cell.com/cell-metabolism/abstract/S1550-4131%2813%2900454-3
10   www.ncbi.nlm.nih.gov/pubmed/18716175
11   www.livinghoney.biz/the-honey-revolution.html
12   http://blog.sethroberts.net/2013/11/05/honey-at-bedtime-improves-sleep
13   www.ncbi.nlm.nih.gov/pubmed/22891435
14   www.ncbi.nlm.nih.gov/pubmed/3508233
15   www.ncbi.nlm.nih.gov/pubmed/20300016
16   www.sciencedirect.com/science/article/pii/003193849090300S
17   www.ncbi.nlm.nih.gov/pmc/articles/PMC2596047/
18   www.ncbi.nlm.nih.gov/pubmed/9760133
19   http://jn.nutrition.org/content/136/2/390.full
20   www.jbc.org/content/285/1/142
21   www.fda.gov/downloads/AdvisoryCommittees/CommitteesMeetingMaterials/MedicalDevices/
MedicalDevicesAdvisoryCommittee/NeurologicalDevicesPanel/UCM291557.pdf
22   www.townsendletter.com/May2010/earthing0510.html
23   www.ncbi.nlm.nih.gov/pubmed/24007813

Chapter 6
1   http://resulb.ulb.ac.be/facs/ism/docs/behaviorBDNF.pdf
2   www.ncbi.nlm.nih.gov/pubmed/21330616
3   www.onlinecjc.ca/article/S0828-282X(13)00258-4/abstract
4   http://care.diabetesjournals.org/content/25/9/1612.short
5   http://cebp.aacrjournals.org/content/15/6/1170.abstract
6   www.nejm.org/doi/full/10.1056/NEJMoa011858
7   www.neurology.org/content/70/19_Part_2/1786.abstract
8   www.ncbi.nlm.nih.gov/pmc/articles/PMC2615833
9   http://europepmc.org/abstract/MED/8164529
10   http://journals.lww.com/acsm-msse/pages/articleviewer.aspx?year=2005&issue=12000&article=
00003&type=abstract
11   http://health.usnews.com/health-news/family-health/brain-and-behavior/articles/2009/05/29/post-
exercise-glow-may-last-12-hours
12   www.ncbi.nlm.nih.gov/pmc/articles/PMC1540458/
13   www.ncbi.nlm.nih.gov/pubmed/12797841
14   www.ncbi.nlm.nih.gov/pubmed/12457419
15   www.ncbi.nlm.nih.gov/pubmed/20837645

Chapter 7
1   http://jn.nutrition.org/content/early/2011/08/26/jn.111.142257.short
2   www.ars.usda.gov/SP2UserFiles/Place/12355000/pdf/0506/usual_nutrient_intake_vitD_ca_phos_
mg_2005-06.pdf
3   www.ars.usda.gov/is/pr/2000/000802.htm
4   www.ncbi.nlm.nih.gov/pubmed/10668486
5   www.ncbi.nlm.nih.gov/pubmed/10022226
6   www.ncbi.nlm.nih.gov/pubmed/19190501
7   www.nytimes.com/2013/06/09/opinion/sunday/dont-take-your-vitamins.html?pagewanted=all
8   http://ajcn.nutrition.org/content/85/1/269S.long
9   http://cdn.marksdailyapple.com/wordpress/wp-content/uploads/2010/12/McAfeeGrassfedbeef
bettern3thanconventionalbeefBJN2011-2.pdf
10   www.ncbi.nlm.nih.gov/pubmed/15537682
11   www.ncbi.nlm.nih.gov/pubmed/12949381
12   www.ncbi.nlm.nih.gov/pmc/articles/PMC1448351
13   www.ncbi.nlm.nih.gov/pubmed/16570523
14   http://ods.od.nih.gov/factsheets/VitaminA-HealthProfessional/

15 www.ars.usda.gov/SP2UserFiles/Place/12355000/pdf/0910/Table_1_NIN_GEN_09.pdf
16 http://lpi.oregonstate.edu/infocenter/vitamins/fa/

Chapter 8

1   www.udel.edu/chem/C465/senior/fall00/Performance1/epinephrine.htm.html
2   Food and Agriculture Organization of the United Nations. *Safety Evaluation of Certain Mycotoxins in Food*. FAO Food and Nutrition Paper 74. Geneva: World Health Organization, 2001.
3   www.ncbi.nlm.nih.gov/pubmed/2721782
4   www.ncbi.nlm.nih.gov/pubmed/7759018
5   www.ncbi.nlm.nih.gov/pubmed/14726276
6   Jorge E. Chavarro, Walter Willett, and Patrick J. Skerrett. *The Fertility Diet*. New York: McGraw-Hill, 2007, p. 73.
7   www.ajog.org/article/S0002-9378(07)02025-X/fulltext
8   www.sciencedirect.com/science/article/pii/S1878764912001155
9   http://ajcn.nutrition.org/content/56/1/148.full.pdf+html
10 www.wholehealthinsider.com/newsletter/nutrient-spotlight-zinc/
11 www.ncbi.nlm.nih.gov/pubmed/7271365
    www.ncbi.nlm.nih.gov/pubmed/1183629
12 www.ncbi.nlm.nih.gov/pubmed/20300016
13 www.ncbi.nlm.nih.gov/pubmed/16097981
14 http://ezinearticles.com/?The-Magic-Bullet-Series:--L-Arginine-and-Fertility!&id=415520
15 www.ncbi.nlm.nih.gov/pubmed/6820754
    www.ncbi.nlm.nih.gov/pubmed/6080242
    www.ncbi.nlm.nih.gov/pubmed/4803052
16 http://jn.nutrition.org/content/137/6/1650S.full
17 http://books.google.com/books?hl=en&lr=&id=7jPRZnISH4wC&oi=fnd&pg=PA175&dq=role+of+glutathione&ots=4JEj7M6pCn&sig=R5mIbIrCT1JyZe7oU8q_xWT5Yik#v=onepage&q=role%20of%20glutathione&f=false
18 www.azcentral.com/health/news/articles/2009/06/13/20090613bloodsugar-spikes-send-testosterone-levels-down.html
19 www.ncbi.nlm.nih.gov/pubmed/15741266?dopt=Abstract
20 http://jap.physiology.org/content/82/1/49
21 www.ncbi.nlm.nih.gov/pubmed/15741266
22 www.ncbi.nlm.nih.gov/pubmed/9029197?dopt=Abstract
23 www.jstor.org/discover/10.2307/4091796?uid=365012351&uid=3739808&uid=2&uid=3&uid=67&uid=308998841&uid=62&uid=3739256&sid=21104509843447
24 http://chej.org/wp-content/uploads/Frequently-Asked-Questions-About-Dioxin-and-Food.pdf

Chapter 9

1   www.ncbi.nlm.nih.gov/pubmed/11988104
2   www.diindolylmethane.org
3   www.ncbi.nlm.nih.gov/pubmed/17652276
4   www.ewg.org/foodnews/summary
5   www.ncbi.nlm.nih.gov/pubmed/20198430
6   www.westonaprice.org/health-topics/nightshades/
7   www.healingcancernaturally.com/garlic-brain-toxin.html
8   www.ncbi.nlm.nih.gov/pubmed/16910057
9   www.inspirationgreen.com/bpa-lined-cans.html
10 http://olivecenter.ucdavis.edu/research/files/oliveoilfinal071410updated.pdf
11 www.motherearthnews.com/real-food/free-range-eggs-zmaz07onzgoe.aspx
12 www.sciencemag.org/content/261/5129/1727
13 www.ewg.org/research/us-gives-seafood-eaters-flawed-advice-on-mercury-contamination-healthy-omega-3s
14 www.ncbi.nlm.nih.gov/pubmed/2818911
15 www.orthomolecular.org/library/jom/1990/pdf/1990-v05n03-p138.pdf
16 www.ncbi.nlm.nih.gov/pubmed/21611739

17 www.ncbi.nlm.nih.gov/pubmed/22555630
18 www.mercola.com/article/soy/avoid_soy.htm
19 www.sciencedirect.com/science/article/pii/S0956713508002442
    www.ncbi.nlm.nih.gov/pubmed/23140362
    www.sciencedirect.com/science/article/pii/S0956713508002442
20 Pusztai A. Dietary lectins are metabolic signals for the gut and modulate immune and hormonal functions. *European Journal of Clinical Nutrition* 1993;47:691–699; Hamid R & Masood A. Dietary lectins as disease causing toxicants. *Pakistan Journal of Nutrition* 2009;3:293–303
21 http://chriskresser.com/raw-milk-reality-is-raw-milk-dangerous
22 http://wageningenacademic.metapress.com/content/5151j377v8v12260/#.U5NbvpSwKJ0
23 Pavelka S. Metabolism of bromide and its interference with the metabolism of iodine. *Physiological Research*. 2004;53 Suppl 1:S81–90

Chapter 10

1   www.ncbi.nlm.nih.gov/pubmed/8212938
2   www.ncbi.nlm.nih.gov/pubmed/10598070
3   www.ncbi.nlm.nih.gov/pubmed/14527787
4   www.ncbi.nlm.nih.gov/pubmed/8480455
5   Martin, Weidenbörner. *Encyclopedia of Food Mycotoxins.* New York: Springer, 2001: p. 177.
6   www.ncbi.nlm.nih.gov/pubmed/11400738
7   http://eur-lex.europa.eu/LexUriServ/LexUriServ.do?uri=OJ:L:2003:168:0033:0038:EN:PDF
8   www.ncbi.nlm.nih.gov/pubmed/7410300
9   www.ncbi.nlm.nih.gov/pubmed/21374488
10 www.ncbi.nlm.nih.gov/pubmed/22864056
11 www.ncbi.nlm.nih.gov/pubmed/21594711 http://www.ncbi.nlm.nih.gov/pubmed/22919440
12 http://care.diabetesjournals.org/content/27/2/436.full
13 http://link.springer.com/chapter/10.1007%2F978-1-62703-167-7_29#page-1
14 www.ncbi.nlm.nih.gov/pubmed/17917911
    www.organicconsumers.org/documents/huber-glyphosates-2009.pdf
15 www.sciencedirect.com/science/article/pii/S095671351300251X
16 www.cholesterol-and-health.com/Goitrogen-Special-Report.html
17 www.ncbi.nlm.nih.gov/pubmed/9149115
18 www.ncbi.nlm.nih.gov/pubmed/10799367
19 www.nature.com/ncb/journal/v11/n11/full/ncb1975.html
20 http://newswise.com/articles/view/539490/
21 www.ncbi.nlm.nih.gov/pubmed/15219719

Chapter 11

1   http://care.diabetesjournals.org/content/27/1/281.full
2   www.ncbi.nlm.nih.gov/pmc/articles/PMC1785201
3   www.ncbi.nlm.nih.gov/pubmed/15771190
    http://aem.asm.org/content/36/2/252.full.pdf
4   www.sciencedirect.com/science/article/pii/0009279795036849
5   www.sciencedaily.com/releases/2007/10/071030102210.htm
6   www.sciencedirect.com/science/article/pii/S2210523914000348
7   www.ncbi.nlm.nih.gov/pubmed/12784390
8   http://onlinelibrary.wiley.com/doi/10.1002/ejlt.201300279/abstract
9   www.sciencedirect.com/science/article/pii/S0926669012004992
10 www.smellandtaste.org/_/index.cfm?action=research.sexual
11 www.orac-info-portal.de/download/ORAC_R2.pdf
12 http://labs.mcdb.lsa.umich.edu/labs/haoxingx/Research_files/Xu,RamseyTRPV3.pdf; Joshi N. The TRPV3 receptor as a pain target: A therapeutic promise or just some more new biology? *Open Drug Discovery Journal* 2010;2:89–97; http://web.archive.org/web/20090624003638/http://vanillaexchange.com/RVCA_Handout.htm www.ncbi.nlm.nih.gov/pubmed/17365147; George A. Burdock. *Fenaroli's Handbook of Flavor Ingredients.* Boca Raton, FL: CRC Press, 2004, p. 277.

13 www.ncbi.nlm.nih.gov/pubmed/20968113
14 www.sciencedirect.com/science/article/pii/S0956713511005640
15 www.ncbi.nlm.nih.gov/pubmed/18539350
16 www.sciencedirect.com/science/article/pii/S0956713511005640
17 www.ncbi.nlm.nih.gov/pubmed/11229375
18 www.ncbi.nlm.nih.gov/m/pubmed/20526682/
19 www.ncbi.nlm.nih.gov/pmc/articles/PMC1285340/
    www.ncbi.nlm.nih.gov/pubmed/16007907
20 www.fda.gov/Food/FoodScienceResearch/LaboratoryMethods/ucm2006949.htm
21 www.ncbi.nlm.nih.gov/pubmed/21994147
    www.sciencedaily.com/releases/2007/02/070215113450.htm
    www.ncbi.nlm.nih.gov/pubmed/11721142
22 www.sciencedirect.com/science/article/pii/S2090123210000330
23 www.ncbi.nlm.nih.gov/pubmed/24436139
24 www.ncbi.nlm.nih.gov/pmc/articles/PMC2892765/#!po=35.7143
25 www.ncbi.nlm.nih.gov/pmc/articles/PMC3856475/
26 www.ncbi.nlm.nih.gov/pubmed/20166324
27 http://nopr.niscair.res.in/bitstream/123456789/12615/1/IJEB%2049%289%29%20689-697.pdf
28 www.intechopen.com/books/soybean-pest-resistance/mycotoxins-in-cereal-and-soybean-based-food-and-feed#T1
29 http://lpi.oregonstate.edu/infocenter/phytochemicals/resveratrol/
30 http://wine.wsu.edu/research-extension/2008/02/mycotoxins/

Chapter 12
1 www.ncbi.nlm.nih.gov/pubmed/1782728
2 www.ncbi.nlm.nih.gov/pubmed/23317342
3 www.aaimedicine.com/jaaim/apr06/hazards.php

Chapter 13
1 www.soilandhealth.org/02/0201hyglibcat/020108.coca.pdf

⬤ ACKNOWLEDGMENTS

This book percolated in my mind for years, but two friends set the wheels in motion to make it happen more quickly than I ever imagined. The first is Rick Rubin, an awe-inspiring guy who, in addition to producing so much of the music that has inspired me in my life, kindly introduced me to a major publisher the day after I mentioned that a book was in the works. The second friend who made this book real is *New York Times* bestselling author JJ Virgin, who runs the Mindshare Collective; she introduced me to her agent Celeste Fine, who became my agent and leapt into action after Rick got the ball rolling. Without their innately helpful way of seeing the world, perhaps this book would still be waiting to be written.

Other wonderful people sought me out and became friends who inspired the work behind this book are guys like world poker champion Nam Le, Third Eye Blind leader Stephan Jenkins, *Superman* and *Arrow* actor Brandon Routh, and Jeremy Piven of *Entourage* fame. Thanks for picking up the phone to let me know how this work has helped you. And sincere thanks to the thousands of Bulletproof blog readers who took the time to reach out and share how their lives have been improved by the practices that are now in this book. You have no idea how much it energizes and inspires me to know that you have been helped by this knowledge!

Tim Ferriss and Peter Sage, thanks for your inspirational work and particularly for your timely advice on the psychology of online trolls. So helpful in the middle of writing this book!

After 15-plus years of collecting ideas from some of the world's most interesting thought leaders and researchers in the anti-aging, medical, biochemistry, psychology, health, and body-building communities and absorbing tens of thousands of pages of research, it's not easy to recognize each person who helped shape this work. Here is my best attempt, and if I've overlooked you, let me know, and please accept my sincere apologies. My gratitude to Dr. Daniel Amen for the groundbreaking brain scan 12 years ago that gave me direction for my biohacking and made me believe that I had the power to change my brain. And to Dr. Helen Irlen for her work explaining how funky orange glasses could turn my brain on in new ways. Dr. Philip Lee Miller, thanks for your pioneering work as an anti-aging physician. Other researchers and authors—some famous, some not— have lit the way along the path of biohacking. Quantified Self leader Seth Roberts, who passed away unexpectedly, leads this list especially because of the conversations we had about carbohydrates and sleep. Others who helped more than they know are Dr. Mary Enig, who tragically passed away during the final stages of writing this book, Dr. Doug McGuff, Rob Faigin, the Westin A. Price Foundation, Dr. Ritchie Shoemaker, Dr. Mark Hyman, Dr. Sara Gottfried, Dr. Pedram Sholjai, Dr. Kate Rheaume-Bleue, Dr. Tom O'Bryan, Roy Dittman, Dr. A.V. Constantini, Dr. Jack Kruse, Mark Sisson for his relentless leadership in the Paleo world, Dr. Kirk Parsley, Dominic D'Agostino, Dr. Terry Wahls, Dr. Alan Christianson, Dr. William Davis, Dr. David Perlmutter, Alberto Villodo, Dr. Grace Liu, Sally Fallon, Dr. Mary Newport, Dr. Oz Garcia, Dr. Stephan Guyenet, Robb Wolf, Vincent Horn, Chris Masterjohn, Dr. Paul Jaminet, Dr. Emily Deans, Aubrey de Grey, Ray Cronise, the indomitable Fat Burning Man himself Abel James, Richard Nikoley, Tater Tim Steele, John Gray, Dr. Mercola, Keith Norris, Denise Minger, Dr. Cate Shanahan, Nora Gedgaudas, gentleman Jimmy Moore, Chris Kresser, Pliny the Elder, and Abelard Lindsay. Gary Taubes's *Good Calories, Bad Calories* is the most elegantly written nonfiction book ever. Thank you. And thanks to Jonathan Bailor for the time you spent compiling 1,000-plus references and writing *The Calorie Myth*. My thanks for the things I've learned from each of you, and I've enjoyed meeting the vast majority of you in person.

Thanks to Michael Fishman, Joe Polish, Dan Sullivan, Michael

Lovitch, Brandon Burchard, Jason Griegnard, Nick Ortner, Jeff Spencer, Napoleon Hill, and Aubrey Marcus for the entrepreneurial coaching and knowledge you've freely shared.

Dan Cox, thanks for your decades of leadership in the coffee business and willingness to talk about it.

Thanks to every one of the 90-plus Bulletproof ambassadors, world-class people who share these practices that work.

Thanks to the incredible people on the Bulletproof team who provide so much motivation and support every single day. Without you, we wouldn't help so many people. Zak, Pascha, and Nikki—thanks for all the extra effort in making this book happen.

Celeste Fine went above and beyond the call of an agent and memorably used the term "spicy meatball" to describe the book proposal. Marisa Vigilante, editor at Rodale, resonated with the Bulletproof vision right away and was a joy to work with. I'll never forget making Bulletproof Coffee for her and the entire amazing team at Rodale in New York City. Jodi Lipper worked with me day and night to get the voice right so it was—I hope—the perfect balance between hands-on how-to info and hard science.

My wife, Dr. Lana, has eaten lots of Bulletproof recipes, and she, along with my kids, Alan and Anna, have pretended to enjoy recipes that weren't really developed yet. I'm grateful for their support and the way they helped to create time for me to write this book. It's also amazing to chat about biohacking over dinner with a Karolinska-trained physician and two little biohackers. Thank you, family. Much love!

The Silicon Valley Health Institute is a 20-year-old nonprofit that's invited more than 100 top experts in aging and human health to share their knowledge with the public. I've been a leader there for about a decade, and the knowledge I aquired there helped to form Bulletproof principles. Without the SVHI board's tireless dedication, this valuable knowledge wouldn't be so accessible. Please join me in thanking them by supporting their nonprofit work at svhi.com. Mike Korek, you're missed. Steve Fowkes, as always, your sage biohacking advice is world-changing, and thanks for your work with SVHI and for your helpful comments on the manuscript. Susan Downs, thank you for your presidency. Larry, Bill, Laurel(s), Dick, Doug, Robert, Sharon, and Phil—thanks for your tireless work over the years to share this precious knowledge.

Thanks also to game changer Lisa Petrison, founder of Paradigm Change, another nonprofit I support; this organization publishes research on mold toxins and human health.

Gratitude to Carrie Simons and her wonderful team at Triple7 PR for helping the world discover this book, and to Ryan Holiday and Tucker Max for doing it even more.

Gratitude is the strongest antidote to stress. I'm truly honored and grateful to be surrounded and supported by so many wonderful people.

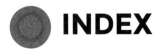 INDEX

Underscored page references indicate sidebars. **Boldface** references indicate charts.